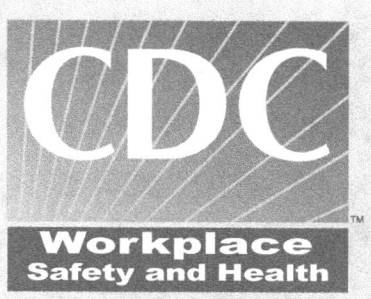

An evaluation of preventive measures at an indium-tin oxide production facility

Kristin J. Cummings, MD, MPH, Eva Suarthana, MD, PhD, Gregory A. Day, PhD, Marcia L. Stanton, BS, Rena Saito, PhD, Kathleen Kreiss, MD

Health Hazard Evaluation Report
HETA 2009-0214-3153
Rhode Island
March 2012

DEPARTMENT OF HEALTH AND HUMAN SERVICES
Centers for Disease Control and Prevention

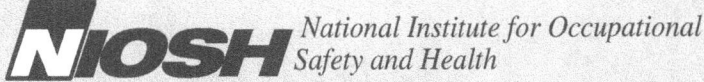

National Institute for Occupational Safety and Health

The employer shall post a copy of this report for a period of 30 calendar days at or near the workplace(s) of affected employees. The employer shall take steps to insure that the posted determinations are not altered, defaced, or covered by other material during such period. [37 FR 23640, November 7, 1972, as amended at 45 FR 2653, January 14, 1980].

CONTENTS

ABBREVIATIONS

APR	air-purifying respirator
ATS	American Thoracic Society
DLCO	diffusing capacity of the lungs for carbon monoxide
EHS	environmental health and safety
ERS	European Respiratory Society
FEV1	forced expiratory volume in one second
FVC	forced vital capacity
GA	general area
GM	geometric mean
GM-CSF	granulocyte-macrophage colony-stimulating factor
HHE	health hazard evaluation
HRCT	high-resolution computed tomography
ILO	International Labour Office
IOM	Institute of Occupational Medicine
ITO	indium-tin oxide
KL-6	Krebs von den Lungen 6
mcg/cm2	micrograms per square centimeter
mcg/L	micrograms per liter
MDC	minimum detectable concentration
mg/m3	milligrams per cubic meter
mL	milliliter
MQC	minimum quantifiable concentration
NIOSH	National Institute for Occupational Safety and Health
NHANES III	Third National Health and Nutrition Examination Survey
OSHA	Occupational Safety and Health Administration
PAPR	powered air-purifying respirator
PPE	personal protective equipment
PR	prevalence ratio
PVC	polyvinyl carbonate
REL	recommended exposure limit
RPP	respiratory protection program

HIGHLIGHTS OF THE NIOSH HEALTH HAZARD EVALUATION

On August 12, 2009, the National Institute for Occupational Safety and Health (NIOSH) received a management request for a health hazard evaluation at an indium-tin oxide production facility in Rhode Island. The company submitted the health hazard evaluation request because of the potential lung toxicity of indium compounds. Two cases of a rare lung disease, pulmonary alveolar proteinosis, occurred among workers at the facility in 2000 (before the current owner purchased the facility) and 2005. The first case occurred in a reclaim worker who died of his lung disease. The second case occurred in an indium-tin oxide department worker who improved with treatment. NIOSH investigators evaluated the preventive measures put in place by the company.

NIOSH provided results and recommendations to the company in an interim report in September 2010 and to employees in workforce presentations in October 2010. Since that time, the company has continued to invest in workplace changes. In addition, the company has met with NIOSH on several occasions to discuss a potential long-term collaboration. This final report reflects the findings reported in the 2010 interim report.

What NIOSH Did

- NIOSH staff toured the facility on April 7-9, 2010.

- We interviewed production managers, safety managers, and current and former workers.

- We interviewed healthcare providers and technicians involved in medical testing conducted for the company.

- We reviewed the company's timeline of workplace changes.

- We reviewed results of air and surface sampling conducted by the company.

- We reviewed personnel information and results of medical testing conducted for the company.

- We interpreted pulmonary function test results using comparisons to U.S. adults.

- We classified chest X-rays for dust-related changes using an international system.

- We measured air concentrations of indium and dust in four work areas.

- We provided feedback to the healthcare providers and technicians to improve the quality of their medical tests.

What NIOSH Found

- Since acquiring the facility in 2002, the company made extensive workplace changes.

- Changes included improved ventilation, isolation of processes, introduction of enclosures on machines, and a comprehensive respiratory protection program.

- From 2004 to 2010, the company conducted 13 air sampling surveys and several surface sampling surveys.

- Indium air levels exceeded 0.1 milligrams per cubic meter throughout the facility and were highest in the refinery and reclaim areas. NIOSH recommended an exposure limit of 0.1 milligrams per cubic meter before indium lung disease was discovered. There is no exposure limit set by regulation.

- Indium air levels did not appear to change over time, although the small number of samples and variations in sampling methods make it hard to compare results.

- The company established a comprehensive medical surveillance program, which included annual blood indium level, spirometry, lung volumes, and diffusing capacity. Chest X-rays were conducted periodically, but not annually.

- Some current and former workers had abnormalities on medical tests suggesting work-related health effects. These include:

    - 21 (50%) had blood indium concentration greater than 5 micrograms per liter after hire. In Japan, doctors have found indium-related lung effects at 3 micrograms per liter and greater.
    - Restriction (small lungs) on spirometry after hire was several times more common than in the general U.S. adult population.
    - Some workers had an abnormal fall in an important lung function measurement during employment.
    - Some workers tested had abnormally low gas exchange after hire.
    - Although test quality was lower than desired, the abnormalities could not be explained by test quality. Abnormalities were as common in good quality tests as in lower quality tests.

- Workers in areas with high indium exposures did not always have more lung abnormalities, suggesting that different types of indium have different risks. For instance:

    - Workers in the refinery had higher levels of indium in the air and in their blood, but few lung abnormalities.

- o Workers in the indium-tin oxide department had lower levels of indium in the air and in their blood, but more lung abnormalities.
- Workers hired from 2007 to 2009 had lower blood indium concentrations and fewer lung function abnormalities than workers hired before 2007, suggesting the company's workplace changes have had a positive impact on exposure and health.

What Managers Can Do

- Control dust migration from production processes.
- Develop procedures to protect workers during upset conditions with potentially high exposures to indium compounds.
- Improve the respiratory protection program including proper use, cleaning, maintenance, and storage of respirators.
- Continue efforts to further lower exposures to indium compounds.
- Continue to monitor workers' health with periodic medical testing.
- Continue to monitor exposures with periodic exposure assessments.
- Enlist NIOSH's assistance to obtain high-quality medical testing and comprehensive assessment of exposure.

What Employees Can Do

- Follow workplace practices intended to reduce exposure to indium compounds.
- Wear personal protective equipment such as a respirator as instructed by your employer.
- Participate in medical testing and air sampling offered by your employer.
- Participate in any medical testing or air sampling offered by NIOSH in the future.
- Report new chest symptoms such as shortness of breath to your employer's health and safety official, the physician conducting medical testing for the company, and your personal physician.
- Call NIOSH at (800) 232-2114 for questions or more information.

SUMMARY

Air levels of indium exceeded the NIOSH recommended exposure limit throughout the facility and workers had abnormalities on medical tests consistent with health effects related to indium compounds. Workers hired more recently had lower blood indium concentrations and fewer lung function abnormalities, suggesting the company's efforts have had a positive impact on exposure and health. We agreed with the company's proactive approach to prevention that includes ongoing workplace improvements and more frequent medical surveillance and made recommendations for additional steps, which could include a long-term collaboration between the company and NIOSH to understand and prevent lung disease related to indium compounds.

On August 12, 2009, the National Institute for Occupational Safety and Health (NIOSH) received a management request for a health hazard evaluation (HHE) at an indium-tin oxide (ITO) production facility in Rhode Island. The company submitted the request because of the potential lung toxicity of indium compounds. The request was for an evaluation of the preventive measures put in place by the company.

To conduct the evaluation, NIOSH staff reviewed and analyzed industrial hygiene and health data provided by the company and healthcare providers, and reviewed supporting documents provided by the company. From April 7 through 9, 2010, we visited the facility to conduct interviews with managers and workers, tour the facility, collect bulk samples, and conduct limited air sampling. We also visited the current pulmonary function laboratory and met with members of the current healthcare provider team at a local hospital.

For historical industrial hygiene data, we grouped samples by type and work area, calculated average values, and examined trends over time. We compared average values to the NIOSH recommended exposure limit (REL) of 0.1 milligrams per cubic meter (mg/m^3). Notably, NIOSH recommended this exposure limit before indium lung disease was discovered. There is no exposure limit set by regulation.

For historical health data, we evaluated test quality, classified results using updated reference equations, calculated frequencies of abnormalities, and examined trends over time. We examined associations between abnormalities and worker characteristics such as employment status, hire date, job title category, blood indium concentration, and estimated indium exposure from the industrial hygiene data.

We found that, since acquiring the facility in 2002, the company made extensive workplace changes. These changes included ventilation enhancements, isolation of processes, introduction of enclosures on machines, a comprehensive respiratory protection program, and a comprehensive medical surveillance program. Records from 13 air sampling surveys that were conducted between 2004 and mid-2010 were provided to NIOSH. We did not find a clear trend in indium concentrations over time. Indium air levels exceeded 0.1 mg/m^3 throughout the facility and were highest in the refinery and reclaim areas.

Records from 57 workers who participated in the medical surveillance program from 2002 to mid-2010 were provided to NIOSH. We found that some current and former workers had abnormalities on medical tests suggesting work-related health effects. For instance, more than half of those tested had blood indium concentration greater than 5 micrograms per liter (mcg/L) after hire. This is important because in Japan, doctors have found indium-related lung effects at 3 mcg/L and greater. Restriction on spirometry after hire and excessive decline during employment in forced expiratory volume in 1 second (FEV_1) (a lung function measurement made using spirometry) were more common than expected. These findings are important because restriction on spirometry can be a sign of lung disease and excessive decline in FEV_1 can be an early marker of lung disease; both have been documented in workers who developed severe lung disease while working with indium compounds. In addition, some workers tested had abnormally low total lung capacity and some had abnormally low diffusing capacity, both of which can be signs of lung disease. Although test quality was lower than desired, the high prevalence of abnormalities could not be explained by test quality. The prevalence of abnormalities was as high in good quality tests as it was in lower quality tests.

Workers in areas with higher indium exposures tended to have fewer lung abnormalities than workers in areas with lower indium exposures. This finding suggests that different types of indium have different health risks and that indium air concentration alone is an inadequate measure of exposure. More sophisticated sampling and analytic methods that account for differences among indium compounds are needed.

Workers hired more recently had lower blood indium concentrations and fewer lung function abnormalities, suggesting the company's efforts have had a positive impact on exposure and health. However, lung function abnormalities among workers hired more recently remained higher than expected, indicating a need for continued exposure reduction measures and ongoing medical surveillance.

In a September 2010 interim report, we recommended further lowering of exposures through engineering controls, keeping indium compounds confined so that they don't contaminate other areas, and proper use, maintenance, and storage of personal protective equipment, including powered air-purifying respirators.

Summary (continued)

We also recommended the use of consistent methods for air sampling, more frequent medical surveillance for newly hired workers, and improvements to the sensitivity and quality of the medical tests included in the surveillance program. Since that time, company officials have met in person with NIOSH officials and staff on two occasions to discuss a potential long-term collaboration to obtain high-quality and commercially unavailable medical testing and comprehensive exposure assessments including an engineering controls evaluation. In November 2011, the company provided NIOSH with an update on workplace changes that had been introduced since 2010 or were planned for the near future. This update made clear that the company anticipated and/or incorporated many of the recommendations we made into its ongoing preventive efforts.

Keywords: NAICS 331419 (Primary Smelting and Refining of Nonferrous Metal [except Copper and Aluminum]), indium, indium oxide, indium tin oxide, interstitial lung disease, pulmonary alveolar proteinosis, lung function tests, spirometry, restriction.

Introduction

On August 12, 2009, NIOSH received a management request for an HHE at an ITO production facility in Rhode Island. The company submitted the HHE request because of the potential lung toxicity of indium compounds. The HHE request was for an evaluation of the preventive measures put in place by the company.

NIOSH provided results and recommendations to the company in an interim report in September 2010 and to employees in workforce presentations in October 2010. Since that time, the company has continued to invest in workplace changes. In addition, the company has met in person with NIOSH staff on two occasions to discuss a potential long-term collaboration. This final report reflects the information contained in the 2010 interim report.

ITO is a sintered material typically consisting of 90% indium oxide (In_2O_3) and 10% tin oxide (SnO_2) [Medvedovski et al. 2008]. ITO is used in the manufacture of such devices as liquid crystal displays, touch panels, solar cells, and architectural glass. In these applications, a thin coating of ITO provides the dual properties of electrical conductivity and optical transparency. Sputtering, a process in which ITO ceramic tiles or "targets" are bombarded with energetic particles that atomize the material, is used to deposit a thin film of ITO on the surface of interest. Exposures to indium compounds (including indium hydroxide [$In(OH)_3$], indium oxide, and ITO) may occur during ITO production, ITO use for the creation of thin films, and reclamation in countries including the United States, Japan, China, Taiwan, and the Republic of Korea.

There is a growing literature indicating adverse health effects related to ITO. From 2003 to 2010, ten cases of symptomatic lung disease, including two deaths, were reported among workers in Japan, the United States, and China [Omae et al. 2011]. The cases occurred throughout the ITO industry, spanning the entire lifecycle of ITO production, use, and reclamation. One case occurred in an indium oxide production facility, where ITO exposure would not be expected. The affected workers were young (median age at diagnosis of 35 years), with relatively short time from hire to diagnosis (median length of 6 years). Symptoms included shortness of breath and cough that did not improve away from work. At an international workshop convened by NIOSH in 2010, expert clinicians identified alveolar proteinosis, cholesterol clefts, cholesterol granulomas, and interstitial fibrosis as common features of the cases; emphysema was noted in more than half of the cases [Cummings et al. 2011].

The workshop participants suggested that exposure to indium compounds causes a new lung disease that may progress from alveolar proteinosis (filling of the lung's air sacs with surfactant, a mixture of protein and lipid) to fibrosis (scarring of the lung tissue) and emphysema (destruction of the lung tissue) [Cummings et al. 2011]. These findings are consistent with the results of animal studies that have demonstrated alveolar proteinosis and pulmonary fibrosis following exposure to a variety of indium compounds including indium oxide and ITO [Leach et al. 1961; National Toxicology Program 2001; Tanaka et al. 2002; Lison et al. 2009; Lison and Delos 2010; Tanaka et al. 2010; Nagano et al. 2011].

Two of the reported cases, including one death, occurred at the Rhode Island ITO production facility that is the subject of this report [Cummings et al. 2010a]. Both affected workers were diagnosed with pulmonary alveolar proteinosis, a rare lung disease that is typically considered of unknown cause (idiopathic), but occasionally occurs in association with other diseases or following occupational dust exposures [Trapnell et al. 2003; Ioachimescu and Kavuru 2006]. In pulmonary alveolar proteinosis, the lung's air sacs fill up with surfactant, a mixture of protein and lipid made by the lung's cells. The excess surfactant impairs gas exchange, the movement of oxygen and carbon dioxide between the lung and the blood. Most patients with pulmonary alveolar proteinosis have symptoms of shortness of breath and cough, although nearly a third of patients in one large series had no symptoms [Trapnell et al. 2003; Ioachimescu and Kavuru 2006; Inoue et al. 2008]. Pulmonary function tests can be normal, but they typically show restrictive pattern on spirometry, mildly reduced lung volumes, and more dramatically reduced diffusing capacity, reflecting the impaired gas exchange [Trapnell et al. 2003]. Chest radiography can show a variety of patterns [Ioachimescu and Kavuru 2006].

The first case of pulmonary alveolar proteinosis at the Rhode Island facility occurred in a reclaim worker and preceded the current owner's 2002 purchase of the facility [Cummings et al. 2010a]. His tasks included crushing used targets and production waste materials by hand or machine and operating a hydrogen-fueled reduction furnace that has since been eliminated. He was hired in 1999, developed symptoms approximately nine months after hire, and was diagnosed with pulmonary alveolar proteinosis in 2000. Despite treatment, he developed radiographic fibrosis (scarring of the lungs) and died of respiratory failure in 2006.

The second case was in a worker in the ITO department, where ITO targets are made from indium oxide and tin oxide powders. His tasks included sanding unfired castings and deburring sintered targets. He was hired in January 2004 and developed intermittent recurrent symptoms of cough, shortness of breath, and chest tightness, approximately six to nine months after hire. He did not seek care for the symptoms, attributing them to the common cold. In September 2005 he experienced a workplace inhalational exposure that led to an evaluation by a pulmonologist and a diagnosis of pulmonary alveolar proteinosis. He did not return to work after the inhalational exposure. He had clinical and radiographic improvement after treatment with whole lung lavage, but remains limited in his activities by his lung disease.

In idiopathic pulmonary alveolar proteinosis, autoantibodies against granulocyte/macrophage colony-stimulating factor (GM-CSF) lead to impaired alveolar macrophage function and decreased surfactant clearance [Trapnell et al. 2003]. In the second case at this facility, autoantibodies against GM-CSF were detected in the worker's blood, raising the possibility of an autoimmune mechanism associated with exposure to indium compounds

[Cummings et al. 2010a; Costabel and Nakata 2010; Cummings et al. 2010b].

There are several reasons to conclude that these two cases of pulmonary alveolar proteinosis were related to exposures occurring during ITO production at this facility. First, there is temporality: exposure preceded disease. Exposure was confirmed in both cases by the detection of indium in lung tissue samples [Cummings et al. 2010a]. Second, pulmonary alveolar proteinosis is quite rare, with an annual incidence of less than 0.5 per million persons [Seymour and Presneill 2002; Inoue et al. 2008]. Thus, the occurrence by chance of two cases in a single facility's small workforce is highly unlikely. Third, there is consistency and specificity between exposure to indium compounds and this rare health outcome. A third case of pulmonary alveolar proteinosis occurred in a Chinese worker exposed to ITO during production of liquid crystal displays for cellular telephones [Xiao et al. 2010]. Furthermore, pathologists participating in the international workshop at NIOSH found histopathological evidence of alveolar proteinosis in nearly all cases of lung disease in workers exposed to indium compounds, regardless of the initial diagnosis [Cummings et al. 2011]. Fourth, there is coherence between epidemiologic and laboratory findings, in that multiple experimental studies have demonstrated alveolar proteinosis in animals exposed to indium compounds [Leach et al. 1961; National Toxicology Program 2001; Lison and Delos 2010; Nagano et al. 2011].

Workplace investigations in Japan have revealed that published cases occurred against a background of subclinical or undiagnosed lung disease in co-workers. At the Japanese ITO production facility in which five of the published cases occurred, 108 current and former workers underwent high resolution computed tomography (HRCT) of the chest; 23 (21%) had significant interstitial changes and 14 (13%) had significant emphysematous changes [Chonan et al. 2007]. Notably, only seven (30%) of the 23 with interstitial changes on HRCT had abnormalities on conventional radiography (chest X-ray). A positive correlation existed between serum indium concentration and both degree of radiographic abnormalities and serum level of the mucin-like glycoprotein Krebs von den Lungen 6 (KL-6), a marker of interstitial lung disease [Kobayashi and Kitamura 1995]. In addition, percent predicted values of total lung capacity and diffusing capacity of the lungs for carbon monoxide (DLCO) decreased with increasing quartile of serum indium. A cross-sectional study of 93 indium-exposed and 93 non-exposed workers in ITO manufacturing and recycling plants in Japan demonstrated exposure-response relationships between serum indium concentrations and serum markers of lung inflammation such as KL-6 and surfactant proteins (SP)-A and SP-D [Hamaguchi et al. 2008].

A subsequent multi-center study of nearly 600 current and former indium workers from 13 indium production, recycling, and research facilities included the workers described by Chonan et al. [2007] and Hamaguchi et al. [2008] [Nakano et al. 2009]. Among current workers, exposure-response relationships between serum indium and KL-6 were observed at serum indium values exceeding 2.9 mcg/L and between serum indium and SP-D at serum indium values exceeding 4.9 mcg/L. Spirometric abnormalities were more common at the highest serum indium concentrations. Similar trends were seen in former workers, who were noted to have exposure-response relationships between serum indium and interstitial abnormalities on HRCT. In addition, concentrations of serum indium and serum markers of lung inflammation were significantly lower in workers who were hired after improvements in the work environment had been implemented, compared to those working before improvements. A more recent study of nine current workers and five former workers who manufactured indium ingots provided evidence that plasma indium concentrations reflect long-term exposure and remain elevated years after exposure cessation [Hoet et al. 2011].

In the years prior to the HHE request, the company in Rhode Island responded proactively to information that exposures occurring during ITO processing may cause lung toxicity. The company initiated periodic air sampling aimed at identifying areas with higher indium exposures, introduced controls in the workplace aimed at reducing airborne exposures, and established a medical surveillance program to closely monitor health indicators in the workforce.

Process Description

The facility has been in operation since the late 1990s under previous ownership and since mid-2002 under the current owner. The following section describes the process as of April 2010.

The facility processes indium metal and tin oxide into ITO ceramic tiles or "targets" used by customers for sputtering applications. In addition, indium metal is reclaimed from used targets that are returned to the facility by customers and from waste materials generated in the production process. Waste materials include cuttings, grindings, rejected castings and targets, and dusts collected from ventilation and recovery systems.

Figure 1 shows the major steps in the production of ITO targets and reclamation of indium. The process begins in the refinery, where indium hydroxide powder is produced from solid indium metal by addition of acid. The indium hydroxide is then converted to indium oxide powder by calcination. In the ITO department, indium oxide and tin oxide along with other compounds are mixed together. The resulting liquid substance ("slip") is cast using a pressurized system into molds for hardening. The castings are dried, undergo limited cutting and sanding, and then are fired. After firing, the now-sintered targets are further ground and cut to customers' specifications in the grinding area. Final deburring is done by hand in the ITO department.

In the reclaim area, spent targets returned from customers and waste materials are converted to indium metal. These materials are first broken down into a powder, transferred via a closed duct system, blended, loaded into crucibles, and heated in a reduction furnace. Molten metal is then cast into ingots. To reclaim additional indium metal, furnace drosses are subjected to further heating followed by chemical dissolution in glass-lined reactors located in the refinery.

Additional information on process controls is found in the Results section under Industrial Hygiene Evaluation: Workplace Changes.

ASSESSMENT

To conduct our evaluation, we collected, reviewed, abstracted, and analyzed industrial hygiene and health data provided by the company and healthcare providers. We also reviewed supporting documents provided by the company. These supporting documents included a list of jobs by production area, a timeline of workplace changes from 2002 to 2009, a current facility map, the Employee Handbook, material safety data sheets, and the facility's written respiratory protection program (RPP). We conducted telephone interviews with company production and environmental health and safety (EHS) managers and healthcare providers.

From April 7 through 9, 2010, we visited the facility. During our visit, we conducted interviews with managers and with current and former workers. These interviews were intended to provide us with a more complete understanding of the process, the workplace changes, and the medical surveillance program. We toured the facility, collected bulk samples, and conducted limited air sampling. We also visited the current pulmonary function laboratory and met with members of the current healthcare provider team at a local hospital. Below are more detailed descriptions of the industrial hygiene and medical evaluations.

Industrial Hygiene Evaluation

Review of Historical Records

On multiple occasions from 2004 to 2010, the company conducted personal and general-area (GA) air monitoring to evaluate exposures to dust (total, inhalable, and respirable) and metals (indium, tin, and tin oxide) in several different work areas, including the refinery, ITO department, grinding area, and reclaim area (Table 1). Samples for airborne total dust were collected using closed-faced, three-piece 37-mm cassettes with either mixed cellulose ester filters or polyvinyl carbonate (PVC) filters. Samples for airborne inhalable and respirable particles were collected using Institute of Occupational Medicine (IOM) stainless steel samplers fitted with a foam dust plug and 10-mm stainless steel cyclones. On one occasion four samples were collected using 4-stage impactors equipped with PVC filters to study particle size distributions in the grinding area, the reclaim area, and the ITO department. Most dust samples were analyzed for indium and some were also analyzed for tin or tin oxide. Surface wipe samples were collected in 2005 and 2007 and were analyzed for indium.

All samples collected by the company were submitted to the same analytical laboratory over the entire time period. The company hired three consultants to conduct exposure assessments in select work areas throughout the facility in 2004, 2008, and 2010; these results were also included in our data analyses.

The analytical methods used by multiple laboratories differed slightly, including associated reporting limits. Some analytical results reported by the laboratories were less than reporting limits (i.e., the minimum masses that could be confidently measured). Our approach for treating these values was to divide values determined for the minimum quantifiable concentrations in air (MQC) by a factor of two. MQCs were calculated by dividing the reporting limit by the volume of air for a given sample. The air samples submitted for gravimetric analysis of total, inhalable, and respirable dust concentrations were analyzed using NIOSH Methods 0500 and 0600 [NIOSH 2003]. Tin and indium concentrations were determined by atomic absorption and/or inductively coupled plasma atomic emission spectrometry using Occupational Safety and Health Administration (OSHA) Methods ID-121 and/or ID-125G [OSHA 2002a, 2002b]. The impactor samples were analyzed using the State of California Method 501 [State of California 1990]. A laboratory used by one consultant in 2008 analyzed samples using in-house methods based on NIOSH Methods 0500, 0600, and 7303.

The company's international EHS manager initially calculated ITO concentrations stoichiometrically by multiplying indium results by 1.86. He later learned that this conversion factor was unreliable and may not accurately represent exposures; therefore, ITO concentrations were not reported after March 2007. As such, we focused our review of sampling data provided by the company on dust measurements (total, inhalable, and respirable) and indium and tin concentrations.

NIOSH Industrial Hygiene Survey

During our visit to the facility, we interviewed workers to obtain more detailed descriptions of their potential exposures during routine work activities, their use of personal protective equipment (PPE), and changes to their job tasks over time. We interviewed the company's international EHS manager who conducted the air sampling to obtain more information about sampling methods, devices, and locations. We also conducted workplace observations, including identification of major tasks involved in each operational area and job title and determination of exposure control methods, such as ventilation, dust suppression by wet-grinding, and use of PPE.

On April 8, 2010 we conducted air sampling at the facility. Our sampling strategy included the collection of samples for determination of concentrations of total dust, respirable dust, indium, and tin. Additionally, we collected airborne dust samples and bulk samples of materials used in various processes throughout the facility for the evaluation of physical and chemical properties.

Full-shift GA air samples were collected from four work areas: refinery, reclaim area (blending room), grinding area, and ITO department. Total dust samples were collected using open-faced, three-piece 37-mm cassette samplers (Omega Specialty Products Division, SKC, Inc., Eighty Four, PA) loaded with PVC filters. Respirable dust samples (i.e., particles equal to or less than ~4 micrometers in diameter) were collected using cyclones (MSA, unknown distributor) mounted onto closed-faced, two-piece, 37-mm cassette samplers loaded with 37-mm, 5-µm pore size, pre-weighed PVC filters. Real-time dust measurements for particles equal to or less than ~10 micrometers in diameter were measured using PersonalDataRAM® model pDR-1000AN/1200 (Thermo Electron Corporation, Franklin, MA). Samples were submitted to the laboratory for gravimetric analysis of total and respirable dusts using NIOSH Methods 0500 and 0600 and for subsequent inductively coupled plasma atomic emission spectrometry analyses of tin and indium using NIOSH Method 7303 [NIOSH 2003]. Additional respirable samples were collected using cyclones mounted onto closed-faced, two-piece, 37-mm cassette samplers loaded with polycarbonate filters for analysis by scanning electron microscopy, but due to technical difficulties, these analyses were not completed and are not reported in the Results section.

Medical Surveillance Evaluation

To describe health trends in the workforce, we reviewed medical surveillance records and chest radiographs of the company's current and former workers. Demographic data (name, date of birth, start date as temporary employee prior to hire by the company, hire date, job title, and termination date) were provided by the company. Medical records were obtained from the following healthcare providers: Clinic A, which conducted medical surveillance for the company until late 2007; Clinic B, which has conducted medical surveillance for the company since late 2007; the laboratories associated with these clinics; and consulting pulmonologists. In some cases, workers have sought care for possible work-related lung disease outside of the surveillance program; such records were reviewed when possible. We included in our analyses the results of questions on respiratory health and the following clinical tests: blood indium level, spirometry, static lung volumes, diffusing capacity, and chest radiography. To clarify the procedures used, we contacted the laboratories that conducted the test of blood indium level and the pulmonary function tests.

Questionnaire

Questions on respiratory health were from OSHA Respirator

Medical Evaluation Questionnaire (available at: http://www.osha.gov/pls/oshaweb/owadisp.show_document?p_table=STANDARDS&p_id=9783) and were self-administered in the context of respirator clearance. We focused on chest symptoms that, while non-specific, could indicate lung disease: shortness of breath, cough, and chest pain.

Blood Indium Level

Blood indium level was determined by the same diagnostic laboratory throughout the surveillance period. The laboratory used inductively coupled plasma mass spectrometry to determine indium concentration. The lowest calibrator used was 5 mcg/L, and the laboratory did not report concentrations below this value. We determined the number of participants who ever had blood indium concentrations greater than or equal to 5 mcg/L during the surveillance period. We calculated the mean and range of indium concentrations of the most recent after-hire tests by worker characteristics. Tests with a value of "none detected" were assigned half of the lowest calibrator value, or 2.5 mcg/L, for these calculations.

Spirometry

Spirometry measures the volume of air that can be inhaled and exhaled. We examined spirometry reports to assign a quality grade on the basis of American Thoracic Society/European Respiratory Society (ATS/ERS) criteria of acceptability and repeatability [Miller et al. 2005]. A grade of "A" represents the highest quality while a grade of "F" represents the lowest quality (Table 2). A grade of A or B indicates a test had at least three curves that were acceptable and repeatable. A grade of C indicates a test had at least two curves that were both acceptable and repeatable. A grade of D indicates a test had one curve that was acceptable. A grade of F indicates a test did not have a curve that was acceptable. According to the ATS/ERS, an unacceptable curve may still be usable (such as for FEV_1) if it has a good start [Miller et al. 2005].

Spirometry reports from Clinic A's laboratory contained sufficient information for grading purposes. Spirometry reports from Clinic B's laboratory contained insufficient information for grading purposes. We requested and received from that laboratory the results of each expiratory effort that comprised the testing session, allowing us to assign a quality grade. We subsequently scored the grades (A=4, B=3, C=2, D=1, and F=0) and calculated the average quality score for each clinic.

We limited our primary analyses to tests with at least one acceptable curve (quality grade of A, B, C, or D). To explore the effect of spirometry quality on interpretation, we also conducted analyses in which we included tests with no acceptable curve (quality grade of F). For spirometric classification, we selected the largest forced vital capacity (FVC) and FEV_1 from the testing session. We compared these volumes to reference values generated from 7,429 asymptomatic participants of the Third National Health and Nutrition Examination Survey (NHANES III) [Hankinson et al. 1999]. We defined obstruction as FEV_1/FVC ratio and FEV_1 below their respective lower limits of normal (5th percentiles) with a normal FVC. We defined a restrictive pattern as normal FEV_1/FVC ratio with FVC below the lower limit of normal. We classified tests with FEV_1/FVC ratio, FEV_1, and FVC below their respective lower limits of normal as having a mixed pattern. Obstruction on spirometry can be seen with conditions such as asthma, emphysema, and chronic bronchitis. A restrictive pattern on spirometry can be seen with conditions such as interstitial lung disease and pulmonary alveolar proteinosis, as well as non-pulmonary conditions such as obesity and neuromuscular disorders. A mixed pattern can be consistent with the presence of both obstructive and restrictive conditions in the tested individual, but more commonly reflects obstruction with hyperinflation in the absence of true restriction [Dykstra et al. 1999]. Among the ten reported cases of lung disease in indium oxide and ITO workers, normal, obstructive, and restrictive patterns occurred [Cummings et al. 2011].

For workers who had more than one spirometry test session, we also examined the change in FEV_1 over time. After adults achieve their maximum lung volume in their mid-20s, they lose an average of about two tablespoons (30 milliliters (mL)) of lung volume every year for the remainder of their lives (if they do not smoke or have other exposures that injure the lungs). We defined excessive decline in FEV_1 as a greater than expected decrease in FEV_1 between any two spirometry tests. The expected decrease in FEV_1 was based on the results of a large study of working males [Wang et al. 2006]. To determine cut-offs for excessive decline, we used the lower limit of normal (5th percentile) values shown in Table 3 [Wang et al. 2006]. Thus, for a test interval of 2 years, a decline greater than 12.2% (6.1% per year times 2 years) would be classified as excessive. We compared the observed to expected proportion of workers with excessive decline in FEV_1 using the chi-square goodness of fit test.

We also examined changes in FEV_1 over time using NIOSH's Spirometry Longitudinal Data Analysis (SPIROLA) Software (http://www.cdc.gov/niosh/topics/spirometry/spirola-software.html). SPIROLA uses the limit of longitudinal decline, which takes into account expected within-person variation in FEV_1 and the duration of follow-up to determine whether or not an individual's decline in FEV_1 may be excessive. After examining the sensitivity of within-person variation settings to detect a fall of 500 mL/year in one of the index cases [Cummings et al. 2011], we used the default setting of 4%. We compared the agreement of the Wang et al. 2006 criteria and SPIROLA by calculating the kappa statistic.

Total Lung Capacity

Determining a lower than expected total lung capacity can confirm lung restriction suggested by a restrictive pattern on spirometry. The pulmonary function laboratory associated with Clinic A did not measure total lung capacity. The pulmonary function laboratory associated with Clinic B measured static lung volumes using helium dilution. We examined static lung volume reports and compared total lung capacity to reference values generated from a stratified random sample of the general population of an entire state [Miller et al. 1983]. We defined restriction as total lung capacity below the lower limit of normal (5th percentile).

Diffusing Capacity

DLCO is a measure of gas transfer in the lungs, and is reduced in interstitial lung diseases, pulmonary alveolar proteinosis, and emphysema. The pulmonary function laboratory associated with Clinic A did not measure diffusing capacity. The pulmonary function laboratory associated with Clinic B has measured DLCO using the single breath technique. We examined diffusing capacity reports for quality on the basis of ATS criteria of acceptability and repeatability [Macintyre et al. 2005]. Diffusing capacity reports from Clinic B's laboratory contained insufficient information to evaluate quality. We requested and received from the laboratory results of each effort that comprised the testing session, allowing us to assess the tests' quality. We compared the average of single breath DLCO values to reference values generated from a stratified random sample of the general population of an entire state [Miller et al. 1983]. We defined low diffusing capacity as DLCO below the lower limit of normal (5th percentile).

Chest Radiography

We classified chest radiographs according to the International Classification of Radiographs of Pneumoconiosis published by the International Labour Office (ILO) [ILO 2002]. This classification system allows physicians to describe the degree of dust-related changes present on a chest radiograph. NIOSH grants B Reader approval to physicians who pass an examination of proficiency in the ILO classification system.

Profusion, or concentration, of small opacities is divided into four major categories (0, 1, 2, and 3), each of which is subdivided into three minor categories, for a total of 12 possible minor profusion categories. We judged category 0 films as having no evidence of dust-related changes (normal), and categories 1 through 3 have increasing degrees of abnormalities consistent with dust-related changes.

The system also includes a description of radiograph quality: Grade 1 (Good, free of technical imperfections or artifacts), Grade 2 (Acceptable, without technical defects or artifacts likely to impair classification), Grade 3 (Acceptable, with technical defects or artifacts but still adequate for classification), and Grade 4 (Unreadable, unacceptable for classification).

Clinic A used traditional film radiography and provided original films to us. Clinic B used digital radiography and provided electronic copies to us. For our analyses, we required at least two independent B readings for each radiograph. As part of the medical surveillance program, radiographs from Clinic A had already undergone one B reading, which we used in our analyses. Radiographs from Clinic B had not been interpreted by a B Reader, as digital standards were not yet available from the ILO. Therefore, for these radiographs, we chose B Readers who were involved in NIOSH's transition to use of digital imaging for detection of pneumoconiosis [NIOSH 2008].

Two B readings of a radiograph were considered to agree when: a) they identified the same major category of small opacity profusion or b) were within one minor category of each other, with the exception of interpretations that spanned the first two major categories (0 and 1), which were considered to disagree (normal and abnormal, respectively). When two B readings agreed, we assigned the B reading with the higher category to the radiograph. Radiographs with B readings that disagreed underwent an additional independent reading by a third B Reader. If two of the three B readings agreed, we used those two B readings and assigned the B reading with the higher category to the radiograph. If all three B readings disagreed, we assigned the B reading with the median category to the radiograph.

Statistical Analyses

The adverse health outcomes were: chest symptoms; abnormal spirometric classification; excessive decline in FEV_1; restriction by static lung volume measurement; low diffusing capacity; and abnormal radiograph. Blood indium concentration of 5 mcg/L or greater served as a surrogate adverse health outcome. We calculated frequencies of adverse health outcomes and examined patterns over time. In addition, we used logistic regression to explore associations between adverse health outcomes and participants' employment status (current versus former workers), hire date (prior to 2007 versus 2007-2009), job title category (Production jobs: ITO grinder, ITO operator, reclaim operator, and refinery operator; other jobs: other jobs with some exposure, other jobs with minimal exposure), and blood indium concentration (below 5 mcg/L versus 5 mcg/L or greater) using contingency tables. We chose 2007 as a cut-point for hire date, as many of the workplace changes were completed by the end of 2006 and blood indium values suggested exposures before and after 2007 differed. The two "other jobs" categories were developed with management input and were meant to reflect relative indium exposure, on the basis of time spent in production and reclamation areas and tasks involved. Other jobs with some exposure were process control technician, laboratory technician, maintenance electrician, maintenance technician, and plant electrician. Other jobs with minimal exposure were mould maker, mould maker assistant, shipper/receiver, production planner/scheduler, health and safety manager, engineering manager, and controller. Management indicated that most workers did not change jobs during employment. In the few cases where a worker had changed jobs, we assigned the worker to the job title with the higher indium exposure for our analyses.

We compared the proportions of the company's workers with obstruction and a restrictive pattern on the most recent spirometry test to the proportion expected from a nationally representative survey. Specifically, we determined prevalence ratios (PRs) of obstruction and restrictive pattern on most recent after-hire spirometry from comparisons with the U.S. adult population prevalence reported in NHANES III [Department of Health and Human Services 1996] using indirect standardization for race (white, black, or Mexican-American), sex, age (17-39 years or 40-69 years), cigarette smoking status (ever or never), and body mass index (normal, overweight, or obese). When smoking status was not available, we made the conservative assumption that the worker was an ever smoker. For our analyses, a PR is the ratio of observed to expected prevalence of obstruction or restrictive pattern. A PR greater than 1 indicates higher than expected prevalence of obstruction or restrictive pattern among the company's workers, while a PR less than 1 indicates lower than expected prevalence of obstruction or restrictive pattern among the company's workers.

All data included in analyses were double-entered into a Microsoft Access database and reviewed for consistency. Analyses were conducted using SAS software Version 9.2 (SAS Institute Inc., Cary, NC). We considered $p \leq 0.05$ to be statistically significant. Identifying information was maintained in accordance with the Federal Privacy Act, 5 U.S.C. § 552a, as amended.

RESULTS

Below we provide the results of our evaluation, which reflect conditions in the facility up to mid-2010. Additional information provided by the company to NIOSH on conditions in the facility after mid-2010 is found at the end of this report.

Industrial Hygiene Evaluation

Workplace Changes

From 2002, when the company acquired the facility, to 2010, when we visited, the company completed various changes in the workplace aimed at exposure reduction. Changes include, but are not limited to, installation of new ventilation filtration devices (i.e., baghouses), process enclosures, and equipment. Prior to the implementation of these changes, the reclaim area utilized a hammer mill and jaw crusher to break up materials before being blended in a cement mixer. Both the hammer mill and jaw crusher were replaced by a different type of mill in an enclosed room. Crushed material from the mill is now transferred via a closed system to a separate blending room. Both rooms (i.e., milling and blending) are kept under negative pressure using a dedicated local exhaust ventilation system. Also in the reclaim area, the company eliminated the use of a hydrogen-fueled reduction furnace.

Other improvements throughout the facility designed to reduce exposures include door flaps and new enclosed grinders in the grinding area, a high-speed door in the refinery, a downdraft table in the inspection room of the ITO department, and tacky mats placed outside of the doors of production and non-production areas. The company also implemented an RPP and associated training. According to the company's written RPP, workers in fusible casting, the grinding area, maintenance, refinery, the reclaim area, and the ITO department are exposed to respiratory hazards including metal fumes, oxide dusts, particulate, and vapors. In the year prior to our visit, the company instituted a zero tolerance policy for non-compliance with respiratory protection requirements. During our evaluation, managers reported that two workers' employment had been terminated on the basis of non-compliance with these requirements.

Historical Industrial Hygiene Sampling

We reviewed the company's air sampling data collected on 13 occasions from 2004 to 2010. A total of 84 personal samples (63 cassettes, 16 IOMs, and 5 cyclones), 30 area samples (25 cassettes, 1 IOM, and 4 impactors), and 19 surface wipe samples were collected over the entire period. It is important to note that many samples of each type were collected for the purpose of estimating dust and/or metal concentrations during short-duration, task-specific activities and that not all sample types were analyzed for both dust and metals. Appendix A contains more detailed information on the historical industrial hygiene sampling data.

Personal Air Sampling

Personal sampling results provided exposure estimates for dust (total, inhalable, and respirable), indium, and tin by work area. All exposure estimates varied throughout the facility.

Dust

A total of 62 total dust cassette samples were collected from 2004 to 2010 in the refinery, reclaim area, grinding area, and ITO department. The majority of samples representative of partial- to full-shift exposures were collected from 2007 to 2009 (n=37). Results indicated that the geometric mean (GM) total dust concentration was highest in the refinery (2.1 mg/m^3; range = 0.68 to 6.4 mg/m^3; n = 4). GM total dust concentrations were lower in the reclaim area (1.2 mg/m^3; range = 0.22 to 5.2 mg/m^3; n = 10) and lowest in the grinding area (0.36 mg/m^3; range = 0.20 to 0.85 mg/m^3; n = 8) and the ITO department (0.24 mg/m^3; range = 0.05 to 0.89 mg/m^3; n = 15).

Inhalable dust samples (i.e., IOM samplers) were not collected in all years or work areas. Two inhalable dust samples were collected in the reclaim area in 2005 (3.8 and 13.7 mg/m^3). In the grinding area, 4 samples collected in 2005 and 2006 ranged from 0.05 mg/m^3 to 1.1 mg/m^3. In the ITO department, 3 inhalable dust samples collected in 2005 and 2006, ranged from 0.4 mg/m^3 to 1.6 mg/m^3.

Respirable dust samples (i.e., cyclones and IOMs) were not collected in all years or work areas. Two cyclone samples were collected in the grinding area in 2005, both resulting in respirable dust concentrations of 0.22 mg/m^3. Nine IOM samples were collected in the reclaim area, grinding area, and ITO department, ranging from 0.05 mg/m^3 to 2.1 mg/m^3. The highest GM respirable dust concentration was in the reclaim area.

Indium

A total of 63 samples were collected for total indium throughout the sampling period but not in all work areas in all years. Results of 38 partial- to full-shift samples indicated that GM total indium concentrations were highest in the refinery (1.5 mg/m^3; range = 0.47 to 3.6 mg/m^3; n = 5), lower in the reclaim area (0.74 mg/m^3; range = 0.06 to 4.0 mg/m^3; n = 10), and lowest in the grinding area (0.17 mg/m^3; range = 0.07 to 0.45 mg/m^3; n = 8) and the ITO department (0.13 mg/m^3; range = 0.03 to 0.59 mg/m^3; n = 15).

Two inhalable indium samples were collected in 2005 from the reclaim area and the grinding area resulting in concentrations of 3.3 mg/m^3 and 0.41 mg/m^3, respectively.

Respirable indium samples (i.e., cyclones n=4 and IOM samplers n=9) were collected in 2005 and 2006. Cyclone samples were collected in 2005 in the reclaim area and the grinding area. The sample collected in the reclaim area resulted in a respirable concentration of 0.27 mg/m^3, and in the grinding area the concentrations ranged from 0.0004 to 0.11 mg/m^3. GM respirable indium concentrations resulting from the 9 IOM samples (reclaim area n= 2, grinding area n=4, ITO department n= 3) ranged from 0.01 to 1.1 mg/m^3, with the highest concentration in the reclaim area (0.35 mg/m^3).

Tin

Forty-two samples were collected for total tin from 2006 to 2010, although not in all work areas. Results of 30 samples were used to evaluate exposures most representative of partial- to full-shift tin exposures. Results indicated that GM total tin concentration was highest in the reclaim area (0.02 mg/m^3; range = 0.002 to 0.12 mg/m^3; n = 8). GM total tin concentrations were lower in the grinding area (0.01 mg/m^3; range = 0.005 to 0.02 mg/m^3; n = 7) and lowest in the ITO department (0.003 mg/m^3; range = 0.0005 to 0.03 mg/m^3; n = 12) and refinery (0.001 mg/m^3; range = 0.0008 to 0.003 mg/m^3; n = 3).

Eight respirable tin samples (i.e., IOM) were collected in 2005 and 2006. Concentrations ranged from 0.001 to 0.89 mg/m^3, with the highest concentrations in the reclaim area.

General-Area Air Sampling

Area sampling results provided estimates of dust (total, inhalable, and respirable), indium, and tin concentrations in three general work areas (reclaim area, grinding area, and ITO department).

Dust

Twenty-five total dust samples (i.e., cassettes) were collected in 2005, 2006, and 2010 in the reclaim area, the grinding area, and the ITO department. Four of the 25 samples were of short duration and were, therefore, not used in our calculation of means. Results indicated that GM total dust concentrations were highest in the reclaim area (1.2 mg/m^3; range = 0.16 to 6.6 mg/m^3; n = 5), lower in the grinding area (0.20 mg/m^3; range = 0.05 to 0.85 mg/m^3; n = 13), and lowest in the ITO department (0.04 mg/m^3; range = 0.02 to 0.14 mg/m^3; n = 3).

Indium

Twenty-five total indium samples were collected in 2005, 2006, and 2010 in the reclaim area, the grinding area, and the ITO department. Again, we excluded four of these samples from our calculation of means because they were short-duration. GM total indium concentrations were highest in the reclaim area (0.45 mg/m^3; range = 0.02 to 4.5 mg/m^3; n = 5), followed by the grinding area (0.03 mg/m^3; range = 0.002 to 0.45 mg/m^3; n = 13), and the ITO department (0.01 mg/m^3; range = 0.009 to 0.02 mg/m^3; n = 3).

Tin

Ten samples were collected for total tin in 2005, 2006, and 2010 in the reclaim area, the grinding area, and the ITO department. One sample was of short duration and was excluded from our calculation of means. The GM total tin concentrations were highest in the reclaim area (0.02 mg/m^3; range = 0.001 to 0.37 mg/m^3; n = 4), lower in the grinding area (0.01 mg/m^3; range = 0.007 to 0.02 mg/m^3; n = 2), and lowest in the ITO department (0.001 mg/m^3; range = 0.0009 to 0.001 mg/m^3; n = 3).

Impactor Sampling

The particle size distribution results from the four samples collected in 2005 using 4-stage cascade impactors varied by operational area. By mass, less than 20% of total airborne particulate was respirable (~ 16% in the grinding area, ~ 10% in the ITO sanding room, and ~ 3% in the reclaim area).

Surface wipe samples

Surface wipe samples were collected in 2005 and 2007 from various surfaces in the facility including tables in the lunch room, lockers in the men's locker room, seats inside workers' personal cars, exhaust ventilation equipment on the roof, and inside respirator masks. Table 4 details the calculated indium concentrations from the surface wipe sample results.

Trends in total indium and total dust concentrations over time

From 2006 through mid-2010, 38 personal air samples were collected in the refinery, the reclaim area, the grinding area, and ITO department to estimate partial- to full-shift total indium exposures. Overall, the GM total indium and total dust concentrations were 0.29 mg/m^3 and 0.52 mg/m^3, respectively.

Refinery

A total of 23 personal samples were collected for total indium in the refinery from 2004 to 2009. The majority of those samples were of short duration (n = 18), with results indicating total indium concentrations of 3.3 mg/m^3 in 2004 (n = 9), 3.4 mg/m^3 in 2006 (n = 2), 0.85 mg/m^3 in 2007 (n = 6), and 0.49 mg/m^3 in 2008 (n = 1). The remaining 5 samples, collected over partial or full shifts, resulted in measurements of 1.2 mg/m^3 in 2007 (n = 3), 1.1 mg/

m^3 in 2008 (n = 1), and 3.6 mg/m^3 in 2009 (n = 1). Although the short-duration total indium measurements appear to indicate a downward trend and the partial- to full-shift measurements appear to indicate an upward trend, the numbers of samples collected by year are too few to discern a clear upward or downward pattern.

Reclaim Area

Eleven personal samples were collected in the reclaim area from 2007 to 2010. Most of those samples were collected over partial to full shifts, results indicating GM total indium concentrations of 1.4 mg/m^3 in 2007 (n = 3), 0.53 mg/m^3 in 2008 (n = 3), 3.3 mg/m^3 in 2009 (n = 2), and 0.1 mg/m^3 in 2010 (n = 2). One short-duration sample, collected in 2008 resulted in a concentration of 0.10 mg/m^3. There is no clear upward or downward trend in these measurements.

Grinding Area

Eleven personal samples were collected in the grinding area from 2006 to 2009. Eight of those samples were collected over partial to full shifts, results indicating GM total indium concentrations of 0.19 mg/m^3 in 2007 (n = 3), 0.17 mg/m^3 in 2008 (n = 1), and 0.15 mg/m^3 in 2009 (n = 4). Three short-duration samples, collected in 2006 and 2007, resulted in measurements of 0.16 mg/m^3 (n = 1) and 0.26 mg/m^3 (n = 2), respectively. There is no clear upward or downward trend in these measurements.

Indium-Tin Oxide Department

Eighteen personal samples were collected in the ITO department from 2006 to 2010. Fifteen of those samples were collected over partial to full shifts, with results indicating GM total indium concentrations of 0.25 mg/m^3 in 2006 (n = 1), 0.13 mg/m^3 in 2007 (n = 5), 0.15 mg/m^3 in 2008 (n = 5), 0.01 mg/m^3 in 2009 (n = 3), and 0.07 mg/m^3 in 2010 (n = 1). Three short-duration samples, all collected in 2007, resulted in a GM concentration of 0.23 mg/m^3. Among these samples, there appears to be a slight downward trend in total indium concentrations across all years.

General area samples were collected in the reclaim area, the grinding area, and the ITO department in 2005, 2006, and 2010. The majority of partial- to full shift samples (18/21) was collected in 2005, which does not allow for evaluation of trends.

Workplace Observations

During our visit to the facility, we observed two saws in the older part of the grinding area that were not enclosed. We did not observe these saws operating. When operated, these saws would be expected to generate a fine mist into the workplace air and cause the operator to come into contact with the cutting fluid, a water-soluble synthetic compound. We also observed that the door separating the sanding room from the casting area in the ITO department was not closed during the sanding of fired tiles.

The company's RPP document contains detailed information on respirator use, cleaning, maintenance, and storage. The company's Employee Handbook makes few references to respiratory protection, but contains an appendix (Appendix 2) that outlines respirator requirements by job operation. We noted some inconsistencies in respirator requirements between the RPP document and Appendix 2 of the Employee Handbook, which may reflect more recent updates to the RPP document. Also, respiratory protection was not included in the Employee Handbook's list of safety equipment furnished by the company.

We observed workers using respirators throughout the facility. These observations included: the use of disposable particulate respirators (dusk masks) in the grinding area and the refinery and by a maintenance worker in the reclaim area; the use of full-face air-purifying respirators in the sanding room and in the mixing area of the ITO department; and the use of powered air-purifying respirators (PAPR) in the reclaim area during material break-down, blending, filling of crucibles, and when skimming dross from the surface of molten metal.

We observed some respirator use practices in the facility that were not consistent with the policies described in the RPP document. While a worker in the mixing area of the ITO department was wearing a full-face air-purifying respirator, workers without respiratory protection were within a distance of less than ten feet. In the reclaim area, workers removed their PAPRs and placed them on an empty crucible before ladling molten metal into casts. This task required one reclaim area worker to stand atop a platform while ladling from an open crucible; this worker did not wear a respirator during this task. Local exhaust ventilation was in place, but appeared insufficient to substantially reduce worker exposure to airborne metal fumes.

We also observed problems with respirator storage, fit, and cleaning. We observed open boxes of particulate respirators placed within work areas. We observed a full-face air-purifying respirator hanging on the door knob to the sanding room. The respirator was later worn by a worker in the same area without being cleaned. In addition, it was apparent that there was not a proper seal between the mask and the worker's face. We were told that respirators are stored in cabinets within each work area, which could lead to contamination of the respirators during storage. We did not observe an area designated for respirator cleaning.

We understood from conversations with company management that the use of latex or nitrile gloves was required in some workplace areas, specifically in the ITO department and in the grinding area. Indeed, we observed some workers in those production areas who wore these types of gloves. In the ITO department, we observed that one worker's glove was torn. Additionally, we learned that some workers wore gloves because of what they described as a tendency for infection to occur when cuts or abrasions on the skin were contaminated by dusts in the workplace.

During our time at the facility, we observed an upset condition in which the closed duct system in the reclaim area was damaged and a cloud of dust outside of the blending room resulted. At the time of the incident, no one in the immediate area was wearing respiratory protection. Company management did not remove employees or themselves from the affected area at the time of the incident despite visible dust in the air and accumulation of dust on the floor. Workers and managers did not don respirators during this event. We were told that this was not the first time that there had been an upset condition in this area.

We were told during interviews with company management and workers that showering is only mandatory for reclaim area workers. However, in the Employee Handbook, item 15 of the plant safety rules list states that all workers in the ITO department, the reclaim area, low melting alloy casting, or the refinery are required to shower at the end of their shift.

NIOSH General Area Air Sampling

Air samples that we collected in April 2010 from the refinery (samplers located beside the sieve machine), ITO department (center of the ITO room), grinding area (near the partially enclosed grinder), and the reclaim area (inside the blending room) revealed total dust concentrations ranging from 0.049 mg/m^3 to 0.272 mg/m^3 and respirable dust concentrations ranging from less than the minimum detectable concentration (MDC) in air to 0.135 mg/m^3 (Table 5). The only total dust concentration above the MQC was in the reclaim area, which was 0.272 mg/m^3; total dust concentrations in all other areas were between the MDC (0.049 – 0.051 mg/m^3) and MQC (0.146 – 0.152 mg/m^3). Respirable dust concentrations in all areas were less than MQC (0.17 – 0.18 mg/m^3) or MDC (0.057 – 0.061 mg/m^3).

Total indium mass concentrations ranged from 0.009 mg/m^3 (ITO department) to 0.136 mg/m^3 (the reclaim area); the only indium mass concentration that exceeded the NIOSH REL for indium (0.1 mg/m^3) was measured in the reclaim area. Respirable indium mass concentrations ranged from 0.002 mg/m^3 (refinery and the grinding area) to 0.042 mg/m^3 (the reclaim area).

Both total and respirable mass concentrations of tin were less than the MDC (< 0.0005 mg/m^3) or the MQC (0.001 mg/m^3) in all areas except the ITO department, where the total and respirable concentrations were 0.003 mg/m^3 and 0.002 mg/m^3, respectively.

Real-time Dust Measurements

In the refinery, we placed the real-time monitor beside the sieve machine, an area isolated from the hallway by a wall and an overhead door. The door remained closed while the operator loaded machines. The real-time dust concentrations (Figure 2) ranged from 0.035 to 0.94 mg/m^3, with an average concentration of 0.07 mg/m^3 (duration = 513 minutes). Peak dust concentrations of approximately 0.45 and 0 94 mg/m^3 were observed while the operator loaded the calcining furnace with indium hydroxide.

In the ITO department, the real-time monitor was located on a work bench in the center of the work area between casting and the sanding room. Approximately five employees worked in this area during the sampling period (509 minutes). The real-time dust concentrations (Figure 3) ranged from 0.018 to 0.092 mg/m^3, with an average of 0.031 mg/m^3. Real-time dust concentrations remained low throughout the sampling period with no notable peaks.

In the grinding area, the real-time monitor was placed on the partially enclosed grinder when sampling began at 7:05AM, but was moved to a work bench located beside the grinder at 11:00 AM. An operator ran the partially enclosed grinder between 11:00AM and 11:20 AM resulting in slightly elevated dust concentrations. Fully enclosed saws were operated in the area during the entire sampling period (496 minutes). The real-time dust concentrations (Figure 4) ranged from 0.033 to 0.202 mg/m^3. The average concentration was 0.068 mg/m^3.

In the reclaim area, the real-time monitor was placed inside the blending room, which was isolated from the hallway by a wall and an overhead door. The door remained closed while operators ran machines inside the room. Real-time dust concentrations (Figure 5) ranged from 0.007 to 8.26 mg/m^3, with an average of 0.168 mg/m^3. The highest concentration was observed when an upset condition occurred at 7:21 AM, resulting in a cloud of dust outside of the blending room. The upset condition was caused when a hole developed at the elbow of the closed transfer system ducting. The operators resumed the process at 8:21AM and completed two batches during the 478 minutes sampling period. There were periodic peak concentrations of approximately 0.25 mg/m^3 every 70 minutes, but due to the lack of observation during the entire sampling period, we cannot identify the task(s) associated with these peaks.

Additional Samples

Table 6 provides information on the 11 bulk samples that we collected for future physicochemical characterization and toxicological studies.

Medical Surveillance Evaluation

The medical surveillance program evolved over time as new diagnostic tests were added. The company's corporate medical director provided input into the program's content. Most recently, the change in providers from Clinic A to Clinic B occurred so that the company could include additional pulmonary function testing (i.e., measurements of total lung capacity and diffusing capacity) not available from Clinic A. Medical surveillance was mandatory for all workers and managers who spend time in production areas and was available to others (such as laboratory workers) who work with indium outside of production areas. Annual surveillance included questions about respiratory health, blood indium level, spirometry, static lung volumes, and diffusing capacity. Chest radiography was conducted periodically, but not annually. The ten workers we interviewed understood that medical surveillance was in place because indium is a potential lung toxin, but none was aware that cases of lung disease (pulmonary alveolar proteinosis), including a fatality, had occurred in his workplace.

Results and recommendations were provided by Clinic B's physician to the individual worker and to the company's regional EHS manager. Abnormal surveillance results could prompt evaluation by a pulmonologist, which could include additional testing. At the time of our evaluation, workers with abnormal pulmonary function test and chest radiograph results were followed with HRCT scans of the chest every six months. When the physician recommended removal of the worker from any work area where he may be exposed to indium, job reassignment was arranged by the company. Reassignment could be to a different job within the same area, if the new job was considered not to have exposure.

A total of 57 workers, all males, were hired by September 30, 2009, participated in some aspect of the medical surveillance program from May 2002 through March 18, 2010, and were included in our analyses. The mean age at hire was 37 years (range 19-56 years). Thirty (53%) were current workers and 27 (47%) were former workers. Thirty-one (54%) were hired prior to 2007 and 26 (46%) from 2007 to 2009. Most (n=52; 91%) participating workers were hired after the current owner's 2002 purchase of the facility. Table 7 shows additional characteristics of the participating workers.

Questionnaire

A total of 70 completed questionnaires from 54 workers had comparable questions on chest symptoms for analysis. Thirty-two workers completed a questionnaire at hire and 2 (6%) reported at least one chest symptom. Four (12%) of 34 workers reported at least one chest symptom after hire. Of 15 workers without reported chest symptoms on the first questionnaire (whether at or after hire) and an available subsequent questionnaire, 2 (13%) reported chest symptoms on the subsequent questionnaire.

Blood Indium Level

The laboratory that conducted the blood indium testing analyzed samples as either plasma (blood without cells but with clotting factors) or serum (blood without cells or clotting factors). Initially, the laboratory used 5 mcg/L as its "reporting value," or cut-off for reporting a concentration of indium. Concentrations of indium below 5 mcg/L were reported as "none detected." In some cases, a reporting value of 10 mcg/L was used, and concentrations of indium below 10 mcg/L were reported as "none detected." In late 2007, the laboratory made an "in-house administrative decision" to change the reporting value to 11 mcg/L. Thus, after 2007, concentrations of indium below 11 mcg/L were reported as "none detected."

We requested that the laboratory provide a measured concentration of indium for all 71 tests with a result of "none detected." In response, the laboratory provided additional results using a reporting value of 5 mcg/L for those tests with a higher reporting value. For 14 tests, the laboratory was not able to provide results using a reporting value below 10 or 11 mcg/L because the samples had been diluted 1:2, the lowest calibrator had been dropped, or the laboratory was not able to find the test in its computer system using the information (name, date of birth, and date of test) we provided. These 14 tests were excluded from our analyses. In total, we identified an additional 10 tests with blood indium level of 5 mcg/L or greater through this request to the laboratory. The remaining 47 tests had a result of "none detected" using the reporting value of 5 mcg/L.

Fifty-one (89%) of the participating workers underwent blood indium testing at least once (including tests done at hire), for a total of 101 tests included in our analyses. Nineteen workers were tested at hire and one (5%) had a blood indium level of 5 mcg/L or greater. The available records did not indicate that this worker had previous indium exposure. Forty-two underwent blood indium testing at least once after hire. Figure 6 shows the mean and range of after-hire blood indium concentrations by year. In 2005, the mean after-hire concentration was 24.1 mcg/L, while in 2009 the mean after-hire concentration was 10.2 mcg/L.

A total of 21 (50%) of 42 workers tested after hire had at least one test showing blood indium level of 5 mcg/L or greater. Figure 7 shows the blood indium concentrations of these 21 workers over time. From 2004 to 2005, there were 5 workers who had substantial increases in blood indium concentration. From 2008 to 2009, the increases that occurred appear more modest.

The proportion with blood indium level of 5 mcg/L or greater and the median concentration varied by hire date and job title (Table 8). Nineteen (70%) of 27 tested workers hired prior to 2007 versus two (13%) of 15 tested workers hired from 2007 to 2009 had at least one test showing a blood indium level of 5 mcg/L or greater after hire. Twenty-one (63%) of 33 tested production workers versus none of 9 tested other workers had at least one test showing a blood indium level of 5 mcg/L or greater after hire. Half of tested current workers and half of tested former workers had a blood indium level of 5 mcg/L or greater after hire. We used the last after-hire blood test to calculate median values. The median blood indium concentration was 11 mcg/L for those hired prior to 2007 versus 2.5 mcg/L for those hired from 2007 to 2009. Refinery operators had the highest median blood indium concentration at 10 mcg/L. Both current and former workers had a median concentration of 3.8 mcg/L.

Spirometry

Clinic A interpreted spirometry tests using reference equations derived from a study of 697 healthy white subjects in Tucson, Arizona [Knudson et al. 1983]. Clinic B interpreted spirometry tests using reference equations derived from a study of 988 healthy white subjects in Northwest Oregon [Morris et al. 1971]. Below we report the results of our interpretations using reference equations derived from NHANES III [Hankinson et al. 1999], which may differ from interpretations using the earlier reference equations.

Fifty-five (97%) of the workers participating in medical surveillance underwent spirometry testing with a total of 138 spirometry tests. We examined the quality of all tests (Table 9). Of 47 spirometry tests conducted by Clinic A, 29 (62%) had A or B grades for both FVC and FEV_1; 5 (11%) had F grades. The average grade was B for both FVC and FEV_1. Of 91 spirometry tests conducted by Clinic B, 16 (18%) had A or B grades for both FVC and FEV_1; 55 (60%) had F grades. The average quality grade was D for both FVC and FEV_1. The most common reason that expiratory curves from Clinic B did not meet acceptability criteria was unsatisfactory exhalation, specifically lack of a volume-time plateau, suggesting that workers were not adequately coached to achieve maximal exhalation.

Incomplete exhalation (evidenced by a lack of a volume–time plateau on the expiratory curve) could lead to underestimation of the FVC and an interpretation of restrictive pattern when lung volumes are truly normal. In examining curves that did not reach a volume-time plateau, we noted that the starts tended to be good, suggesting the tests were usable [Miller et al. 2005]. In addition, the curves' slopes generally were not steep at the point of termination, indicating that the amount of additional volume that would have been recorded had a volume-time plateau been achieved was probably quite small. Thus, while these tests did not meet the strict quality criteria, our impression was that they were unlikely to grossly underestimate the FVC and thereby unlikely to lead to generally false interpretation of restrictive pattern in workers with normal lung volumes. To evaluate the effect of spirometry quality on interpretation, we examined quality grade and interpretation using the most recent after-hire spirometry tests (Table 10). When we limited the analysis to the 13 workers with good spirometry quality (FEV_1 and FVC of grade A or B), 5 (38%) had a restrictive pattern. When we included 3 workers with grade C quality, 5/16 (31%) had a restrictive pattern. When we included 7 workers with grade D quality, 9/23 (39%) had a restrictive pattern. When we included 22 workers with grade F quality, 14/45 (31%) had a restrictive pattern. Thus, the inclusion of tests with poor spirometry quality does not appear to have overestimated the prevalence of restrictive pattern among workers at this facility. In order to achieve a more representative analysis with larger numbers, rather than be limited to an analysis of a much smaller and less representative group, we present below the results of our interpretation of all spirometry tests regardless of quality, unless otherwise noted.

Twenty-eight workers were tested at hire: 5 (18%) of these tests showed a restrictive pattern, 2 (7%) showed obstruction, and 21 (75%) were normal. Forty-five workers underwent spirometry testing at least once after hire: 18 (40%) of these workers had at least one test showing a restrictive pattern after hire, 5(11%) had at least one test showing obstruction, and one (2%) had at least one test showing a mixed pattern. The proportion with a restrictive pattern on spirometry after hire varied by employment status and hire date (Table 11). Nine (33%) current workers and 9 (50%) former workers had at least one test showing a restrictive pattern after hire. Thirteen (52%) workers hired prior to 2007 and five (25%) workers hired from 2007 to 2009 had at least one test showing a restrictive pattern after hire. Thirteen (38%) of 34 production workers, 4 (57%) of 7 other workers with some exposure, and 1 (25%) of 4 other workers with minimal exposure had at least one test showing a restrictive pattern after hire.

Table 12 shows the PRs (observed/expected) of restrictive pattern on spirometry comparing this company's workers with the U.S. adult population. When all spirometry tests regardless of quality were included in the analysis, the prevalence of a restrictive pattern on spirometry among this company's workers was 4.0 times the corresponding prevalence for the U.S. adult population, a statistically significant difference. When results were restricted to acceptable quality spirometry (FEV_1 and FVC of grade A, B, C, or D), the prevalence of a restrictive pattern on spirometry among this company's workers was 5.3 times the corresponding prevalence for the U.S. adult population, also a statistically significant difference. When the results were restricted to good quality spirometry (FEV_1 and FVC of grade A or B), the prevalence of a restrictive pattern on spirometry among this company's workers was 5.6 times the corresponding prevalence for the U.S. adult population, also a statistically significant difference. Thus, the inclusion of tests with poor spirometry quality does not appear to have overestimated the PRs of restrictive pattern. For these analyses, we assumed 12 workers for whom smoking status was unavailable were ever smokers. PRs were similar when we assumed these 12 workers were non-smokers. PRs for obstruction demonstrated that the prevalence of obstruction among the company's workers was not elevated compared to the corresponding prevalence for the U.S. adult population.

Eighteen (33%) workers were tested at hire and during employment. Comparisons of spirometry interpretation from their at-hire and most recent spirometry tests (regardless of quality) are shown in Table 13. Of 13 workers with a normal interpretation at hire, 1 (8%) had obstruction and 3 (23%) had a restrictive pattern on the most recent spirometry. All 4 of these workers also had an excessive decline in FEV_1, resulting in abnormality. When the analyses were restricted to acceptable quality spirometry (FEV_1 of grade A, B, C, or D), a comparison of FEV_1 from the baseline and last spirometry tests was possible for 7 workers. Of 5 workers with normal interpretation at baseline, 1 (20%) showed a restrictive pattern on the last test. This worker also showed an excessive decline in FEV_1. Of two workers with a restrictive pattern at baseline, one had a restrictive pattern and one had a normal result on the last test. When the analyses were restricted to good quality spirometry (FEV_1 of grade A or B), the comparison of FEV_1 from the baseline and last spirometry tests was possible for only 3 workers. Of 2 workers with normal interpretation at baseline, 1 had a restrictive pattern and 1 had a normal result on the last test. The worker with the restrictive pattern on the last test also showed an excessive decline in FEV_1. One worker had a restrictive pattern at baseline but a normal result on the last test.

Of 41 workers with at least two tests, 26 workers had normal interpretation on their first test (whether at or after hire). Two of these 26 (8%) had obstruction and 4 (15%) had a restrictive pattern on their last test. All 6 of these workers also had an excessive decline in FEV_1, resulting in abnormality. When the analyses were restricted to acceptable quality spirometry (FEV_1 of grade A, B, C, or D), a comparison of FEV_1 from the baseline and last spirometry tests was possible for 18 workers. Of 11 workers with a normal result on the first test, 2 (18%) showed a restrictive pattern on the last test. Both workers also had an excessive decline in FEV_1. Of 7 workers with a restrictive pattern on the first test, four had a restrictive pattern on the last test. One of these 4 had an excessive decline in FEV_1. When the analyses were restricted to good quality spirometry (FEV_1 of grade A or B), the comparison of FEV_1 from the first and last spirometry tests was possible for 8 workers. Two (40%) of 5 workers with normal interpretation on their first test had a restrictive pattern on their last test.

We evaluated the presence of excessive decline in FEV_1 in 41 workers with at least two tests, where the first test was done either at hire or during employment (Tables 14a; Table 14b excludes five workers with spirometric interpretation of obstruction). A total of 12 (29%) ever had an excessive decline in FEV_1, significantly higher than expected (p<0.0001). Eight (30%) of 27 current and 4 (29%) of 14 former workers ever had an excessive decline in FEV_1. Based on job category, 4 (57%) of 7 ITO grinders and 5 (33%) of 15 ITO operators ever had an excessive decline in FEV_1. When the analyses were restricted to spirometry with good FVC and FEV_1 quality ("A" or "B" grade), there were 5 (50%) of 10 workers who ever had an excessive decline in FEV_1. When we included workers with grade C quality, 5/11 (46%) had an excessive decline in FEV_1. When we included workers with grade D quality, 5/22 (23%) had an excessive decline in FEV_1. Thus, the inclusion of tests with poor spirometry quality does not appear to have overestimated the prevalence of excessive decline in FEV_1.

SPIROLA identified 10 (24%) workers with excessive decline in FEV_1 during employment on the basis of limit of longitudinal decline criteria. Agreement between the two methods was 85% (kappa=0.63).

Total Lung Capacity

Lung volume testing was initiated in late 2007 by Clinic B. Thirty-seven (65%) of the workers participating in medical surveillance underwent lung volume testing with a total of 91 tests. Although we did not conduct a formal quality review, we noted that many of the lung volume test reports indicated an inadequate helium equilibration time of 0.00 minutes, calling into question the quality of the tests. However, when we inquired about this issue, the laboratory informed us that the information on the reports was incorrect, and the helium equilibration time was generally 2 to 3 minutes.

Clinic B interpreted lung volume tests using reference equations of Goldman and Becklake [1959]. Below we report the results of our interpretations using reference equations of Miller et al. [1983], which may differ from interpretations using the earlier reference equations.

One (8%) of 12 workers tested at hire had a low total lung capacity, indicating restriction. Thirty-five (61%) of the 57 workers participating in medical surveillance underwent at least one lung volume test after hire (Table 15). Of these 35, 8 (23%) were interpreted as ever having a low total lung capacity, indicating restriction. A total of 7 (26%) of 27 current workers and 1 (13%) of 8 former workers ever had a low total lung capacity after hire. A total of 3 (25%) of 12 ITO operators and 2 (40%) of 5 of reclaim operators ever had a low total lung capacity after hire.

The occurrence of new cases of low total lung capacity was evaluated in 33 workers with at least two total lung capacity measurements. Of 27 workers with normal total lung capacity on the first test (whether at or after hire), 2 (7%) had low total lung capacity on the last test. Of 6 workers with a low total lung capacity on the first test (whether at or after hire), 4 (67%) had a low total lung capacity on the last test (including the one with low total lung capacity at hire) and 2 (33%) had a normal total lung capacity on the last test.

Diffusing Capacity

Diffusing capacity testing was initiated in late 2007 by clinic B.

Thirty-seven (65%) of the 57 workers participating in medical surveillance underwent diffusing capacity testing with a total of 91 tests. We excluded one test effort due to poor quality.

Clinic B interpreted diffusing capacity tests using reference equations of Gaensler and Wright [1966]. Below we report the results of our interpretations using reference equations of Miller et al. [1983], which may differ from interpretations using the earlier reference equations.

All of 12 workers tested at hire showed a normal diffusing capacity. Thirty-five (61%) workers underwent at least one diffusing capacity test after hire (Table 16). Of these, 8 (23%) were interpreted as ever having low DLCO, indicating low diffusing capacity. A total of 5 (19%) of 27 current workers and 3 (38%) of 8 former workers ever had low DLCO after hire, indicating low diffusing capacity. A total of 2 (33%) of 6 of ITO grinders and 4 (33%) of 12 ITO operators ever had low DLCO after hire, indicating low diffusing capacity. Tests interpreted as having low diffusing capacity had acceptable curves and met repeatability criteria.

The occurrence of new cases of low diffusing capacity was evaluated in 33 workers with at least two diffusing capacity tests. Of 28 workers with normal diffusing capacity on their first test (whether at or after hire), 2 (7%) had a low diffusing capacity on their last test. Of 5 workers with a low diffusing capacity on the first test, 3 (60%) had a low diffusing capacity on the last test and 2 (40%) had a normal diffusing capacity on the last test.

Co-occurrence of Lung Function Abnormalities

Table 17a shows that 7 (44%) of 16 workers with a restrictive pattern on spirometry also had an excessive decline in FEV_1, in comparison to 5 (20%) of 25 workers without a restrictive pattern on spirometry. Likewise, 7 (88%) of 12 workers with an excessive decline in FEV_1 had a restrictive pattern on spirometry, in comparison to 9 (31%) of 29 workers without an excessive decline in FEV_1. Table 17b shows the results when five workers with spirometric obstruction are excluded.

Table 17c shows that 7 (58%) of 12 workers with a restrictive pattern on spirometry had low total lung capacity, indicating restriction, in comparison to 1 (4%) of 23 workers without a restrictive pattern on spirometry. Likewise, 7 (88%) of 8 workers with low total lung capacity, indicating restriction, had a restrictive pattern on spirometry, in comparison to 5 (19%) of 27 without low total lung capacity.

Table 17d shows that 3 (25%) of 12 workers with restrictive pattern on spirometry had a low diffusing capacity, in comparison to 5 (22%) of 23 workers without a restrictive pattern on spirometry. Likewise, 3 (38%) of 8 workers with a low diffusing capacity had a restrictive pattern on spirometry, in comparison to 9 (33%) of 27 workers without a low diffusing capacity.

Table 17e shows that 2 (25%) of 8 workers with low total lung capacity, indicating restriction, had a low diffusing capacity, in comparison to 6 (22%) of 27 without a low total lung capacity. Likewise, 2 (25%) of 8 workers with a low diffusing capacity had low total lung capacity, indicating restriction, in comparison to 6 (22%) of 27 workers without a low diffusing capacity.

Chest Radiography

Forty-six (81%) of the 57 workers who participated in medical surveillance had chest radiography as part of medical surveillance with a total of 64 tests. Of 31 chest radiographs conducted by Clinic A, 18 (58%) were Grade 1, 11 (36%) were Grade 2, and 2 (6%) were Grade 3 quality. Of 33 chest radiographs conducted by Clinic B, none was Grade 1, 23 (70%) were Grade 2, and 10 (30%) were Grade 3 quality. The most common reasons that radiographs from Clinic B did not meet Grade 1 criteria were the presence of artifact and problems with exposure.

None of 25 chest radiographs done at hire was abnormal. Twenty-eight (48%) workers had chest radiography at least once after hire with a total of 39 tests. Two (7%) workers who had normal baseline chest radiographs had subsequent abnormal chest radiographs after hire that were consistent with pneumoconiosis. Both workers were reclaim operators hired prior to 2007 and had blood indium concentrations greater than 5 mcg/L after hire.

In addition, two former workers had diffuse abnormalities on chest radiographs done after hire outside of the formal surveillance program. The first was an ITO grinder who had an excessive decline in FEV_1 of 700 mL in one year, five years after hire. His chest radiograph was interpreted by a radiologist as showing multiple reticulo-nodular densities throughout both lungs. He was evaluated by a pulmonologist, who thought that the abnormalities were likely caused by exposures at work. The pulmonologist noted near complete resolution of the abnormalities over the course of one month. We were unable to contact this former worker or obtain subsequent imaging studies. The second was the ITO operator who was ultimately diagnosed with pulmonary alveolar proteinosis.

Referral to Pulmonologist

Five (9%) of the 57 workers who participated in medical surveillance were referred to a pulmonologist as a result of abnormal findings on medical surveillance tests. The worker who developed pulmonary alveolar proteinosis was referred to a pulmonologist on account of an acute inhalational injury, rather than his abnormal medical surveillance results.

Exposure-Response Relationship

We used logistic regression to examine the association between a group of five adverse health effects ever after hire (restrictive pattern on spirometry, excessive decline in FEV_1, low total lung capacity, low diffusing capacity, and abnormal chest radiograph) and worker characteristics. Adverse health effects were not associated with employment status (p=0.35). Adverse health effects were significantly less common in workers hired more recently (2007-2009) than in workers hired before 2007 (p<0.01). Adverse health effects appeared to vary with job title, but these differences were not statistically significant (p=0.16), likely due to small numbers in subsets. Adverse health effects tended to be more common in workers with blood indium level of 5 mcg/L or greater, but these differences were not statistically significant (p=0.07). Table 18 summarizes estimates of exposure and adverse health effects by job and is discussed in detail in the Discussion section of this report.

DISCUSSION

Context

Lung disease related to indium compounds is an emerging health issue about which many questions remain. For instance, we know little about the exposure-response relationship. It appears that not only ITO but also indium oxide can cause lung disease, and perhaps other indium compounds encountered in the ITO industry. What characteristics of the responsible compounds are important, such as particle size, form (gas, vapor, mist, or dust), and concentration? Is cumulative or peak exposure relevant?

DISCUSSION (CONTINUED)

What influences do work processes such as mixing, spraying, and grinding have? We also have limited knowledge of the disease process. Exposures during ITO production appear to lead to one disease that can evolve from pulmonary alveolar proteinosis to fibrosis and emphysema. Why did some workers present early in employment and others later? Why have some cases been marked by inexorable progression and others by some degree of stabilization? What role does autoimmunity play? Is the process reversible with a reduction in exposure? For how long does indium persist in the body even after work exposure to indium compounds ceases, putting workers at risk through an immunologic or toxic mechanism?

Given our limited and evolving understanding of lung disease related to indium compounds including ITO, a precautionary approach to prevention is warranted. This company appropriately introduced a preventive program aimed at reducing exposures throughout the facility. We found that the workplace changes have been extensive: ventilation improvements, machine enclosures, isolation and automation of processes, and required use of respiratory protection in some areas. Many of these changes were completed by the end of 2006, but others (particularly in the reclaim area) were more recent, and additional improvements have occurred (see below) and are planned. Indeed, it was clear from our interactions with managers that, despite the many changes that have already been introduced, the company sees exposure reduction as an ongoing process. The ultimate goal of exposure control is to limit potential risk of adverse health effects.

Medical Surveillance Evaluation

To monitor workers for adverse health effects, the company developed a medical surveillance program that is one of the most comprehensive we have reviewed. This medical surveillance program reflects the company's substantial commitment to worker health.

Our analyses of the medical surveillance data indicated that many workers had abnormalities on medical tests. We found that half of the workers had blood indium levels above 5 mcg/L. This level is concerning because a cut-off of 3 mcg/L has been suggested for preventing early effects of indium on the lungs [Nakano et al. 2009]. We also found that more than 30% of the workers had a restrictive pattern on spirometry, which was at least 4 times more common than expected from comparisons with the U.S. adult population. Furthermore, about a quarter of the workers had an abnormal fall in lung volume (FEV_1) over time, beyond what would be expected from normal aging. In addition, about a quarter each had low total lung capacity and low diffusing capacity after hire, when we would expect no more than 5% of healthy non-smokers to have such abnormalities.

What could cause this apparent disproportionate burden of lung function abnormalities in these workers? A restrictive pattern on spirometry can be seen with certain lung diseases and other conditions (such as obesity and neuromuscular disorders) that cause the lungs to be smaller than normal. In some cases, obesity may have been responsible for an individual worker's restrictive pattern on spirometry. Yet our analyses accounted for the effects of weight and still found that a restrictive pattern was more common than expected. Furthermore, 12 workers with a restrictive pattern on spirometry underwent testing for total lung capacity (Table 17b). Of these, 7 (58%) had a low total lung capacity, indicating that the lungs were smaller than expected. If representative of all the workers with restrictive pattern on spirometry, this finding suggests that more than half of all of the workers with a restrictive pattern on spirometry truly had abnormally small lungs (restriction).

Another possible explanation is that low test quality caused abnormal results. We did find that spirometry quality was much lower than desired; ideally, all tests would have three acceptable curves and be repeatable within 150 mL (quality grade A or B) [Miller et al. 2005]. However, in our analysis of the spirometry data, we did not find any evidence that low test quality influenced the proportion with restrictive pattern. Good quality spirometry had a similar proportion of tests with restrictive pattern as low quality spirometry. Low quality spirometry could also have influenced detection of abnormal fall in the volume of air blown out in the first second of the test (FEV_1) over time. However, the FEV_1 is unlikely to be affected by the most common quality issue we observed (lack of volume-time plateau). We did not conduct a formal quality review for the test of total lung capacity. We found that all but one of the workers with low total lung capacity had a restrictive pattern on spirometry (Table 17b), which is about what we would expect from a good quality test of total lung capacity. We reviewed the diffusing capacity tests for quality, and did not encounter quality issues in those tests that indicated a low diffusing capacity. Thus, we cannot readily invoke low test quality as an obvious explanation for the apparent disproportionate burden of lung function abnormalities among these workers.

Smoking is a well-known cause of lung disease. However, we cannot attribute the burden of lung function abnormalities in these workers to smoking. Smoking-related lung disease takes decades to develop, and these workers were relatively young, with a mean age less than 40 years at hire. In addition, unless very severe, smoking-related lung disease would be expected to result in obstruction (not a restrictive pattern) on spirometry, and would not be expected to cause low total lung capacity. In some individual workers with a low diffusing capacity but normal or elevated total lung capacity, smoking-related emphysema could explain the low diffusing capacity. However, for the vast majority of workers with a low diffusing capacity, smoking-related emphysema is not a plausible explanation due to young age, low total lung capacity, or relatively few years of smoking.

Asthma is a common lung disease that could affect a relatively young group of workers. People with asthma have either a normal pattern, obstruction, or a mixed pattern (not solely a restrictive pattern) on spirometry. Thus, asthma does not account for our restrictive pattern findings. Worsening asthma could lead to an abnormal fall in FEV_1 over time. However, the majority (7 of 12, or 58%) of the workers with an excessive decline in FEV_1 had a restrictive pattern on spirometry, which suggests their abnormal fall in FEV_1 was not related to asthma. Furthermore, asthma does not cause low total lung capacity or low diffusing capacity, so cannot explain these abnormalities.

Another possible explanation for the burden of lung function abnormalities in these workers is that they represent pre-existing conditions in workers. We did not find convincing evidence for pre-existing restrictive lung disease. Lung function abnormalities consistent with restrictive lung disease were far less common among workers tested at hire than among workers tested after hire. For instance, the prevalence of a restrictive pattern on spirometry was 18% in those tested at hire and 31% in those tested after hire; the prevalence of low total lung capacity was 8% in those tested at hire and 17% in those tested after hire; and the prevalence of low diffusing capacity was 0% in those tested at hire and 17% in those tested after hire. Although not all workers were tested at hire, the available evidence indicates that the majority of the lung function abnormalities were not present at hire, but appeared to develop during employment.

There are several reasons to conclude that the burden of lung function abnormalities in these workers is primarily related to the workers' common exposure to indium compounds. First, there is a temporal relationship to exposure in that most abnormalities followed employment. Lung function abnormalities were more common after hire than at hire. Excessive declines in FEV_1 occurred during employment, after exposure to indium compounds began. Second, the types of abnormalities we observed (restrictive pattern, abnormal fall in FEV_1, low total lung capacity, and low diffusing capacity) are all consistent with the reported health effects of indium compounds. Third, both blood indium levels above 5 mcg/L and lung function abnormalities tended to be less common in workers hired more recently (2007 to 2009). This relationship is what we would expect if exposure to indium compounds both increases indium in the blood and causes damage to the lungs. We conclude that past exposures to indium compounds were high enough to cause adverse health effects. The proportions of lung function abnormalities in workers hired more recently (2007 to 2009) were lower than those among workers hired before 2007, suggesting the company's workplace changes had a positive impact on exposure and health. However, the abnormalities among workers hired more recently generally remained elevated (for instance, see Table 12). If these abnormalities were related to exposure to indium compounds, as the evidence suggests, then more recent exposures to indium compounds were still not low enough to prevent adverse health effects.

How low must indium exposures be to prevent lung health effects? The existing NIOSH REL of 0.1 mg/m³ [NIOSH 2005] for indium and indium compounds was introduced in the 1980s. The REL thus predates the reports of interstitial lung disease and pulmonary alveolar proteinosis in the ITO industry. As such, it should not be assumed to be protective against these diseases. While the Japanese experience with lung disease in ITO production workers has been the most extensive, industrial hygiene evaluations either have been limited [Chonan et al. 2007] or not pursued [Hamaguchi et al. 2008; Nakano et al. 2009] in Japanese studies. The Japanese government recently introduced a standard for respirable indium of 3×10^{-4} mg/m³ on the basis of animal studies of indium oxide and ITO toxicity [Ministry of Health, Labor, and Welfare, 2010]. Whether this level will be protective remains to be determined.

In the absence of a known protective exposure limit, guidance can be derived from observed health outcomes among the exposed workforce. In effect, a safe exposure level is one at which workers do not develop adverse health outcomes that are reasonably related to indium compounds. This company's medical surveillance program could be a means to determine a safe indium exposure limit, by examining cohorts by date of hire as the company continues to lower indium exposures.

Industrial Hygiene Evaluation

Our review of the historical sampling data found that GM total indium concentrations in the partial- to full-shift personal air samples ranged from 0.13 (ITO department) to 1.45 mg/m^3 (refinery), without an observed decline over time. Among the partial- to full-shift area air samples, GM total indium concentrations ranged from .01 (ITO department) to 4.5 mg/m^3 (reclaim). The GM total indium concentration in grinding was 0.03 mg/m^3. Chonan et al. (2007) reported an indium concentration of 0.05 mg/m^3 in the grinding area of a facility with affected workers. The area air sampling that we conducted on April 8, 2010 showed indium concentrations ranging from 0.009 mg/m^3 (ITO department) to 0.136 mg/m^3 (reclaim area). These concentrations suggest lower exposures than in the past, but may also reflect differences in sampling strategy and technique (such as our reliance on GA samples, which may underestimate exposures compared to personal samples) that make direct comparisons challenging. With only four GA air samples, our results are unlikely to be representative of personal exposures.

The workers who developed pulmonary alveolar proteinosis while at the Rhode Island facility developed chest symptoms within a year of employment [Cummings et al. 2010a]. The second worker with pulmonary alveolar proteinosis was followed with spirometry and had an excessive decline in FEV$_1$ of 500 mL in his first year of employment. While little is known about the relevant exposure characteristics, the rapid development of disease suggests the possibility that peak concentrations (rather than cumulative exposures) may be important.

The real-time dust monitoring that we conducted provides potentially crucial peak exposure information that is not captured by full-shift measurements. Real-time monitoring can be used to determine the ranges of dust concentrations throughout the facility, to evaluate the effectiveness of local exhaust ventilation systems, to evaluate work practices, and to identify potential sources of upset conditions. For instance, the real-time dust monitoring results from a sample collected from inside the blending room in reclaim suggested that the highest indium concentration occurred when a hole developed at the elbow of the closed transfer system ducting. This ducting was external to the blending room. We did not collect samples outside the room, but would expect the dust and indium concentrations to be higher than inside the enclosed room during such an event. Although workers mandatorily used PAPRs while inside the blending room when the process was operational, respirators were neither required nor worn when outside the blending room during this upset condition. In light of this upset condition, the company should consider implementing respiratory protection measures to be utilized during upset conditions to minimize peak exposures. One preventive measure to consider is the installation of a secondary containment system to capture process emissions due to failure of the primary system. Use of real-time monitoring is one way to identify peak exposures that cannot be identified using conventional sampling methods.

The historical surface wipe samples indicated that indium was detected on multiple surfaces, including inside respirators, on the lunchroom table, in the locker room, and inside workers' cars (Table 4). These results indicate that indium migration may create exposure opportunities and that exposure to indium compounds may occur in unexpected ways. For example, settled indium-containing dust on surfaces may become re-suspended in air, may contaminate workers' skin and clothing, and may be transported off-site. Two surface wipe samples collected from the tops of lockers in the men's locker room demonstrated the presence of indium-containing dust, with indium concentrations of 80.2 micrograms per square centimeter (mcg/cm^2) and 101.4 mcg/cm^2. Five surface wipe samples collected from the seats of workers' personal cars demonstrated the presence of indium-containing dust; the highest concentration of 13.7 mcg/cm^2 was measured in a grinding area worker's car. The presence of indium-containing dust in workers' cars suggests that workers are taking these dusts home with them, thereby potentially putting non-workers (i.e., family members) at risk. During our walk-through of the facility, we toured the locker room, lunchroom, and break areas. We understand that these areas are cleaned by contract housekeeping staff and that company uniforms are picked up once a week for laundering off-site. During our visit, we observed that uniforms were overflowing from the laundry container onto the floor, which could also contribute to dust contamination and migration.

Exposure-Response Relationship

As noted previously, the exposure-response relationship between indium compounds and lung disease is poorly understood at this time. Existing animal studies, case reports, and cross-sectional investigations of workplaces provide some guidance. Animal studies demonstrate that ITO is particularly toxic [Lison et al. 2009], but also implicate other indium compounds, including indium oxide [Leach et al. 1961; American Conference of Governmental Industrial Hygienists 2001; National Toxicology Program 2001; Tanaka et al. 2002; Lison et al. 2009; Lison and Delos 2010; Nagano et al. 2011]. Early case reports of lung disease in ITO production workers focused on the task of wet surface grinding [Homma et al. 2003; Homma et al. 2005], but more recent reports describe health effects in workers who carried out other tasks as well, such as other ITO production tasks and tasks related to reclamation [Chonan et al. 2007; Cummings et al. 2010a]. In addition, a recent case report describes lung disease (specifically pulmonary alveolar proteinosis) in a worker exposed to ITO during the production of cellular telephones [Xiao et al. 2010]. Finally, one case occurred in an indium oxide production facility, where ITO exposure would not be expected [Cummings et al. 2011]. Such observations suggest that while risk may not be uniform throughout a facility, it is unlikely to be limited to a certain compound or production process.

We attempted to explore the exposure-response relationship by examining exposures and health outcomes by job (Table 18). We found that indium exposure (as measured by total indium in historical personal air samples) was highest for refinery operators, followed by reclaim operators. ITO grinders and ITO operators had similar, lower indium exposures. Estimates were not possible for workers in other jobs with some exposure or other jobs with minimal exposure. Another potential measure of exposure is blood indium level. We found that blood indium levels of 5 mcg/L or greater were common in production workers but not in other jobs considered to have lower exposure to indium. Indeed, more than half of the workers in each production job title, but none of the other workers, had blood indium levels of 5 mcg/L or greater. Estimates of exposure to indium thus seem to create two groups: Higher (refinery operator, reclaim operator, ITO grinder, ITO operator) and Lower (other some exposure, other minimal exposure). Using a blood test with a lower detection limit might enable refinement of exposure categories.

Adverse health outcomes were most common in ITO operators and reclaim operators, intermediate in ITO grinders, and least common in refinery operators. For each measure of lung function, 20 to nearly 50% of ITO operators and reclaim operators had abnormalities. Furthermore, all four abnormal chest radiographs and both known cases of pulmonary alveolar proteinosis were found among workers in these two job titles. In contrast, with the exception of one worker with a restrictive pattern on spirometry, refinery operators had no lung function abnormalities. Workers in other jobs with minimal exposure also had few lung function abnormalities. Abnormalities were more common among those in other jobs with some exposure. Indeed, more than half of the workers in other jobs with some exposure had a restrictive pattern on spirometry and half had low total lung capacity, comparable to the findings in ITO operators and reclaim operators. Estimates of adverse health response (low lung function results, abnormalities on chest radiography, and occurrence of pulmonary alveolar proteinosis) thus seem to suggest two groups that are somewhat different from those suggested by estimates of exposure: Higher (ITO operators, reclaim operators, other some exposure) and Lower (ITO grinders, refinery operators, other minimal exposure).

If, as we demonstrated earlier, exposure to indium compounds is likely to be the primary cause of the adverse health outcomes in these workers, why do we see this apparent discrepancy between surrogates for exposure and health response? There are several possible explanations related to the limitations of the data we analyzed. First, the exposure data may not accurately reflect true exposure. The historical air samples were not collected in a systematic way to make estimates of exposure by job title. Rather, they were primarily intended to identify areas with higher indium concentrations and assess the local effects of workplace changes. Furthermore, estimates were not available for non-production jobs. In addition, the blood indium level reporting value of 5 mcg/L may not be an appropriate cut-off for determining exposure. In Japan, lung damage on chest imaging (HRCT) was observed in former indium workers with a serum indium level of 3.0-4.9 mcg/L [Nakano et al. 2009]. At the Rhode Island facility, the second worker with pulmonary alveolar proteinosis had a blood indium level less than the reporting value of 5 mcg/L more than a year into employment, yet had measureable indium in a lung tissue specimen [Cummings et al. 2010a]. Thus, although measured blood indium levels suggest that workers in non-production jobs did not have exposure to indium compounds, that conclusion may not be correct. Second, the data may not accurately reflect response. Lung function tests and chest radiography were not always conducted at hire, limiting our ability to differentiate abnormalities that developed during employment (plausibly work-related) from abnormalities present at hire (not work-related). Given the small numbers of workers in each job category, one or two workers with pre-employment abnormalities or with spirometry results influenced by poor quality testing could obscure true associations between exposure and health outcomes. Third, despite our efforts to accurately assign workers to job titles and job titles to categories, some misclassification may have occurred due to limited information on individual work histories and job exposure characteristics.

Another consideration is that the healthy worker effect may have played a role [Li and Sung 1999]. The healthy worker effect occurs when workers who develop work-related symptoms or disease transfer within a plant away from a particular work area or leave a plant entirely. Workers remaining behind in that particular work area or plant are generally less susceptible and may appear healthier than the general population or workers in other work areas of the plant. The availability of medical records after workers left employment was limited, so it is possible that some workers developed adverse health effects during employment but left employment before undergoing annual medical surveillance testing, or developed adverse health effects after employment.

It is also possible that the data do accurately reflect both exposure and response, but that the exposure-response relationship is more complex than can be understood from the available information. For instance, the role of autoimmunity in lung disease related to indium compounds is not clear. A recent report from Japan indicates that if autoimmunity played a role in the second case of indium lung disease at this plant, the mechanism of indium compounds' toxicity is not exclusively autoimmune [Masuko et al. 2011]. Lung disease with an autoimmune mechanism might occur at lower exposure thresholds or with peak exposures that are not well reflected by the historical air sampling results or blood indium levels. Indeed, there is evidence from other immune-mediated occupational lung diseases that peak exposures are most relevant to disease development [Leroyer et al. 1998; Klees and Ott 2000; Jacobs et al. 2008]. Lung disease that is not autoimmune might occur with higher exposures or in relation to cumulative exposures that build up a body burden of indium over time. Despite these limitations, it is notable that refinery operators had among the lowest rates of lung function abnormalities, despite the fact that most had blood indium levels of 5mcg/L or greater. The indium compounds in the refinery are distinct from those found elsewhere in the facility, and perhaps different indium compounds vary in their interactions with the lungs and the blood. However, it is also possible that the small number of refinery operators led us to miss an exposure-response relationship that would have been evident with a larger group of refinery operators.

The difference in blood indium levels by hire date is also notable. In general, indium appears to persist in the blood long after exposure. One Japanese study looked at former indium workers who had left employment an average of 5 years before testing. The mean serum indium concentration was 9.63 mcg/L, which was similar to the mean concentration among current workers in the study of 8.35 mcg/L [Nakano et al. 2009]. A more recent study of nine current workers and five former workers who manufactured indium ingots provided evidence that plasma indium concentrations reflect long-term exposure and remain elevated years after exposure cessation [Hoet et al. 2011]. Thus, for the workers with long tenure, blood indium levels may reflect a legacy of past exposure that does not speak to current workplace conditions. By examining blood indium levels by hire date, we attempted to differentiate between past and more recent conditions. We found that 70% of workers hired before 2007 but just 13% of those hired since 2007 had blood indium levels of 5 mcg/L or greater. Some of this difference may reflect differential testing. A total of 87% of workers participating in medical surveillance and hired before 2007 versus 62% of workers participating in medical surveillance and hired since 2007 have undergone blood indium testing after hire. It is also possible that this gap will close somewhat in the future, as the more recently hired workers spend more time at the facility. The change in the laboratory's reporting value from 5 to 11 mcg/L also may have had an impact, but we accounted for this change to the extent possible by requesting indium concentrations regardless of reporting value used. Thus, the difference in blood indium levels by hire date appears real and suggests that exposures have indeed fallen in recent years.

Detection of Adverse Health Effects

We found that some aspects of the medical surveillance program may limit the company's ability to detect lung disease at an early stage. The use of respiratory questions in the context of respirator clearance (a prerequisite for job performance) may lead to under-reporting of chest symptoms within the surveillance program. Furthermore, respiratory symptoms may appear relatively late in the disease process, after a point at which abnormalities in lung function could be detected. Thus it is unlikely that questions on respiratory symptoms, particularly in the context of medical clearance for respirator use, can effectively detect lung disease at an early stage.

The laboratory that conducts blood indium testing currently uses a reporting value of 11 mcg/L, and has never reported concentrations below 5 mcg/L. Given that Japanese authors have reported health effects at concentrations as low as 3 mcg/L [Nakano et al. 2009], a reporting value of 5 or 11 mcg/L seems inappropriately high.

In addition, we found that the quality of spirometry tests conducted by Clinic B was low. In most cases, curves did not meet acceptability criteria because of lack of a volume-time plateau, which could underestimate FVC and lead to an interpretation of restrictive pattern in the absence of true restriction. Our sensitivity analyses did not demonstrate any obvious relationship between quality score and prevalence of a restrictive pattern, suggesting that the low quality did not generally influence interpretations of restrictive pattern.

Yet spirometry quality has important implications when following workers' lung function over time. A primary goal of monitoring indium-exposed workers with spirometry should be to detect changes in lung function before a substantial loss in lung function has occurred (i.e., typically before a restrictive or obstructive pattern has developed), so that steps can be taken to prevent further decline. For workers who already have abnormal spirometry (restriction, obstruction, or mixed pattern), longitudinal spirometry can be used to determine if lung function is declining further. Detecting losses in lung function over time requires high quality spirometry characterized by low variability from measurement errors [Hnizdo et al. 2010].

The use of outdated reference equations also is a concern. Clinic A and Clinic B interpreted spirometry using reference equations from small, homogeneous, geographically isolated populations that were studied decades ago and are unlikely to be representative of the company's workers [Knudson et al. 1983; Morris et al. 1971]. The ATS [Pellegrino et al. 2005] recommends the use of spirometry reference equations derived from NHANES III, a nationally representative sample of more than 7000 subjects that included whites, blacks, and Hispanics [Hankinson et al. 1999]. In the case of medical surveillance of ITO industry workers, a particular concern is that the older equations are less likely than those derived from NHANES III to identify a restrictive pattern [Sood et al. 2007; Collen et al. 2008; Collen et al. 2010]. Thus the use of reference equations from Knudson et al. 1983 and Morris et al. 1971 may underestimate the number of workers with spirometric abnormalities consistent with toxicity from indium compounds and limit the ability to detect lung disease at an early stage. We have similar concerns about the reference equations from the 1950s and 1960s used by Clinic B for the lung volume and diffusing capacity tests. The staff at Clinic B's pulmonary function laboratory indicated that they were in the process of obtaining new test equipment, which may address many of these issues.

Another issue is that standard chest radiographs are likely to be an insensitive tool for detecting early changes in the lungs. In the Japanese study that found abnormalities consistent with interstitial lung disease on HRCT scan of the chest in 23 (21%) of 108 ITO production workers, just 7 of these had abnormalities on chest radiograph [Chonan 2007]. Lower quality chest radiography, as we found with Clinic B, will only make detection of abnormalities more error-prone.

The frequency of testing must be considered in the context of what is known about disease latency and progression. Both of the workers at this facility who developed pulmonary alveolar proteinosis noted symptoms during the first year of employment. More frequent testing early in employment could facilitate early disease detection, and has been used in other workplace settings where some workers may be more susceptible to another occupational lung disease [Cummings et al. 2007]. More frequent testing of newly employed workers also serves to provide earlier feedback on the effectiveness of new workplace changes.

Finally, there may be other biomarkers that would be useful for early detection of lung disease in these workers. Japanese authors reported strong associations between markers of lung inflammation that can be detected in the blood and serum indium concentration

[Nakano et al. 2009]. Autoantibodies to GM-CSF may also have a role in detecting pulmonary alveolar proteinosis at an early stage. Indeed, 30% of patients with pulmonary alveolar proteinosis were asymptomatic at diagnosis but had detectable autoantibodies to GM-CSF in one study [Inoue et al. 2008]. Currently, the test for autoantibodies to GM-CSF is available only on a research basis.

Response to Adverse Health Effects

Despite the large number of workers with lung function abnormalities, few workers were referred to a pulmonologist for further diagnostic evaluation. It appears that referral has been triggered in the past when abnormalities were found on multiple tests, including abnormal chest radiograph. This approach may be reasonable in the primary care setting, when the probability of rare lung disease is low and hazardous exposures are absent. However, in the context of medical surveillance for an emerging occupational lung disease, a lower threshold for referral is appropriate. For example, the worker who developed pulmonary alveolar proteinosis had a 500 mL fall in FEV_1 nearly one year before his eventual diagnosis, which was prompted not by medical surveillance but by an inhalational exposure. Earlier referral to a pulmonologist may have led to a more prompt diagnosis and treatment, potentially altering the course of his disease.

One powerful diagnostic tool available to a pulmonologist is HRCT of the chest. As noted earlier, the Japanese have demonstrated that HRCT is a more sensitive tool than chest radiography for detecting abnormalities that may be related to indium exposure [Chonan et al. 2007]. Notably, abnormalities on HRCT consistent with interstitial lung disease were common (27% prevalence) among former workers who had been away from exposure to indium compounds for an average of 5 years [Nakano et al. 2009]. Thus there is reason to expect that abnormalities related to indium compounds, once detected, may persist and do not need to be reconfirmed. The benefit of repeated, frequent use of HRCT (such as twice yearly) in this setting is unlikely to outweigh the associated radiation risk incurred [Smith-Bindman 2010]. An alternative would be more frequent use of good quality pulmonary function tests to evaluate for changes over time.

How should this company manage workers with abnormalities on pulmonary function tests or radiography that are consistent with lung disease related to indium compounds? Given our limited

DISCUSSION (CONTINUED)

understanding of the exposure-response relationship, minimizing these workers' exposures through job reassignment and use of personal protective equipment would be prudent. Although our analyses indicate that there are few locations and jobs at the facility that are without indium exposure, the jobs we categorized as other jobs with minimal exposure (mould maker, mould maker assistant, shipper/receiver, production planner/scheduler, health and safety manager, engineering manager, and controller) appear to be lower-risk from the perspective both of indium exposure and adverse health outcomes. For workers with abnormalities consistent with lung disease related to indium compounds who cannot be relocated to one of these jobs, full-time use of a PAPR (with assigned protection factor of 1000) would be warranted throughout the facility.

Open communication with workers about the risks and uncertainties of indium exposure is vital. The company's efforts to share information about animal toxicity studies and Japanese reports of lung disease were laudable and were reflected in workers' general knowledge about indium toxicity. However, the interviews we conducted with workers demonstrated that they were not aware of the occurrence of cases of lung disease in their own workplace. The sharing of such information can motivate an improved safety culture, including enhanced compliance with respirator use policies.

Future Steps

Since the release of the NIOSH interim report in 2010, the company has met in person with NIOSH on two occasions to discuss a potential long-term collaboration to determine the effectiveness of ongoing and newly introduced preventive measures. Such a collaboration could include high quality medical testing and research blood tests (KL-6, GM-CSF auto-antibodies) of the current workforce conducted by NIOSH and a comprehensive industrial hygiene evaluation to characterize representative full-shift and real-time exposures and better differentiate between exposures to various indium compounds.

CONCLUSIONS

In response to information that exposures occurring during ITO processing may cause lung toxicity, the company has made extensive workplace changes and established a comprehensive medical surveillance program. We found that historical records of air sampling for indium did not demonstrate a clear trend in indium concentrations over time. We also found that some workers have abnormalities on medical tests suggesting work-related health effects. Workers hired more recently had lower blood indium concentrations and fewer lung function abnormalities, suggesting the company's efforts have had a positive impact on exposure and health. Nonetheless, given our limited understanding of both the exposure-response relationship and the disease process, a precautionary approach that emphasizes further lowering of indium exposures and enhanced monitoring of adverse health outcomes among exposed workers is prudent.

RECOMMENDATIONS

These recommendations were made in the interim report that was provided to the company in September 2010. Following these recommendations, we include information provided by the company in November 2011 on the status of its workplace changes. From this updated information, it is clear that the company anticipated and/or incorporated many of the recommendations we made into its ongoing preventive efforts.

The hierarchy of controls approach is traditionally recommended as a strategy for creating a more healthful workplace. In this hierarchy, the preferred approach is to first eliminate hazardous materials or processes and install engineering controls to reduce exposure or shield workers. Until such controls are in place, or if they are not effective or feasible, administrative measures and/or personal protective equipment may be needed.

In the case of an emerging occupational health issue such as potentially fatal lung disease related to indium compounds, we agree with the company's comprehensive approach that has included multiple aspects of the hierarchy to reduce the risk of lung toxicity during ITO processing. We recommend these following additional steps as further improvements:

Engineering Controls

Engineering controls reduce exposures to workers by removing the hazard from the process or placing a barrier between the hazard and the worker. Engineering controls can be very effective at protecting workers.

1. Separation and isolation of areas (migration control)

   - Clean and non-clean areas in the locker room should be separated.

   - The company should continue to monitor the effectiveness of the local exhaust ventilation in the reclaim area.

   - Given the upset condition we observed and the risk of its reoccurrence, routine observation and maintenance of the duct system in the reclaim area should be instituted. A back-up system to prevent the release of indium-containing dusts in the event of damage to the duct system should be considered.

2. Some tasks in the reclaim area that involve metal fumes are carried out with limited ventilation controls and without respiratory protection. Given our limited understanding of the toxicity of different forms of indium, monitoring of exposures to metal fumes during tasks in the reclaim area and providing additional ventilation controls (and respiratory protection, see below) would be prudent.

Administrative Controls

Administrative controls are management-dictated work practices and policies to reduce or prevent exposures to workplace hazards. The effectiveness of administrative changes in work practices for controlling workplace hazards is dependent on management commitment and worker acceptance. Regular monitoring and reinforcement is necessary to ensure that control policies and procedures are not circumvented in the name of convenience or production.

1. Housekeeping practices should be improved to minimize surface contamination in locker rooms, lunchroom, break areas, and production areas.

2. Efforts to control the migration of contamination within individual work areas should include attention to work practices that prevent migration via hands, clothing, and shoes. Efforts to control the migration of contamination

between work areas should include limiting the transfer of tools and equipment. To avoid contamination of workers' personal vehicles and home environments, showering at the end of the shift should be required for all indium-exposed workers.

3. A section on emergency procedures should be added to the Employee Handbook detailing procedures for the immediate evacuation and isolation of work areas in the event of an upset condition. Workers with clean-up responsibilities should be provided with the necessary personal protective equipment, including but not limited to: respirators, eye and hearing protection, and chemical-protective clothing and gloves. Other workers should not re-enter the area(s) until an "all clear" signal has been given.

4. Hazard communication – Workers need to be aware of the risks of occupational exposure to indium during ITO production and reclamation. We agree with the company's recent efforts to share information about the toxicity of ITO and other indium compounds with workers and encourage the company to explore ways that results of ongoing medical surveillance could be communicated to workers on a regular (such as annual) basis. In addition, we recommend that a brief section on indium toxicity be added to the Employee Handbook. This section should define what indium compounds are, describe the potential hazards of handling and processing indium-containing compounds, and outline current information on exposure opportunities (i.e., inhalation, skin contact). This information may further motivate workers to recognize and avoid potential hazards associated with indium and reinforce the need for proper use of PPE, including respiratory protection.

5. Whenever possible, workers with any otherwise unexplained abnormalities consistent with indium-related lung disease should be relocated to other jobs with minimal exposure. Such abnormalities include an excessive decline in FEV_1 or the development of any of the following: a restrictive pattern on spirometry, low total lung capacity, low diffusing capacity, or dust-related changes on chest radiograph or HRCT. As a precaution, relocation should occur whether a definitive diagnosis has or has not been made (see Medical Surveillance below).

Personal Protective Equipment

PPE is the least effective means for controlling worker exposures. Proper use of PPE requires a comprehensive program and calls for a high level of worker involvement and commitment to be effective. The use of PPE requires the choice of the appropriate equipment to reduce the hazard and the development of supporting programs such as training, change-out schedules, and medical assessment if needed.

1. Our observations of the use and storage of respirators by the company's workers indicate that workers need additional and ongoing training on the proper use, cleaning, maintenance, and storage of respiratory protection. This information should be included in the Employee Handbook.

2. Respiratory protection should be added to the list in the Employee Handbook of safety equipment to be furnished by the company.

3. The Respiratory Protection Program document and the Employee Handbook should be modified to assure that they both provide consistent information on respirator type and filter replacements requirements by job operation.

4. The company should provide a proper location for the cleaning, maintenance, and storage of respirators.

   - Proper cleaning and disinfection of respirators requires a clean area where the respirator can be disassembled, washed with a mild detergent in warm water, rinsed in clean warm water, and allowed to air dry in a clean area prior to reassembly according to manufacturer recommendations. Given the work environment, respirators should be cleaned at the end of each shift and disinfected at least weekly.

   - Cabinets for respirator storage should be located outside of the work area, to prevent contamination.

1. The role of skin exposure in causing indium-related lung disease is unknown. Nevertheless, workers should be encouraged to comply with the company's current glove use policy.

RECOMMENDATIONS
(CONTINUED)

2. Respiratory protection should be worn in the reclaim area during tasks with exposure to metal fumes.

3. In work areas where PAPRs are not currently used, PAPRs with assigned protection factor of 1000 should be made available to workers desiring a higher level of protection than required by the company.

Industrial Hygiene Sampling

Our review of historical sampling data revealed that sampling methods and reporting procedures for dust, indium, and tin changed over time, which made evaluation of trends challenging. These changes may have reflected the company's need to answer different questions with different surveys. We recognize that in the future, novel sampling strategies may be needed to address new questions. Nonetheless, the inclusion in each survey of consistent methods for sampling and reporting dust and metal concentrations would facilitate monitoring of concentrations in workplace air over time and determination of trends. This exposure assessment may be critical in the future determination of health-protective exposure guidance.

Medical Surveillance

Our review of the medical surveillance program revealed that the current medical surveillance program is comprehensive. However, the program has had some problems with quality testing that have gone unrecognized, and the sensitivity of the blood indium test that has been used is limited. The following recommendations are primarily intended to improve (rather than expand) the current program, to allow the company to better detect possible occupational lung disease at an early stage.

1. Frequency of testing – For newly hired workers, we recommend more frequent medical surveillance using lung function testing during the first year of employment. Until quality issues are resolved, testing of newly hired workers should occur at hire and at 3, 6, and 12 months of employment. Once high-quality testing is in place, it may be reasonable to eliminate testing at 3 months.

2. Blood indium – Blood indium testing should be done

by a laboratory that is able to accurately determine the concentration of indium in blood using a limit of detection far lower than 5 mcg/L. The method used in the Japanese studies has a limit of detection of 0.1 mcg/L [Nakano et al. 2009]. We understand that the only commercial clinical laboratory providing blood indium testing in the US is (at NIOSH's request) currently updating its methodology to improve the limit of detection.

3. Spirometry quality – Spirometry quality improvement is crucial for optimally valid interpretation of test results, particularly for longitudinal assessment of lung function. We found the most common reason that the FEV_1 and FVC curves from Clinic B did not meet acceptability criteria was unsatisfactory exhalation, specifically lack of plateau, which could be readily improved through technician training and ongoing quality feedback from a supervising pulmonologist or audits by an independent third party. Following the release of the interim report, we reviewed a series of spirometry tests conducted by Clinic B's technician and provided feedback for further improvement. Additional feedback and, if warranted and desired by the technician, training, could be provided by NIOSH as part of a future collaboration with the company.

4. Longitudinal spirometry – Currently Clinic B only assesses the spirometry abnormality classifications (i.e , restrictive, obstructive, or mixed pattern). Given that spirometry is conducted serially and at least annually, we recommend longitudinal assessment of the lung function measurement using rate of decline over time (i.e., excessive decline in FEV_1) for early identification of at-risk workers. [Hnizdo et al. 2010]. Spirometry Longitudinal Data Analysis (SPIROLA) software is an easy-to-use visual and quantitative tool intended to assist the healthcare provider in monitoring and interpreting computerized longitudinal spirometry data for individuals as well as for a group. SPIROLA software can be downloaded for free from the NIOSH website and easily installed (http://www.cdc.gov/niosh/topics/spirometry/spirola html).

5. Reference equations – The reference equations for spirometry, lung volume testing, and diffusing capacity testing currently used by Clinic B's pulmonary function laboratory are outdated. We recommend reference equations derived from NHANES III [Hankinson et al.

1999] for spirometry and from a sample of the general population of an entire state [Miller et al. 1983] for total lung capacity and diffusing capacity measurements. The staff at Clinic B's pulmonary function laboratory indicated that they were in the process of obtaining new test equipment, which may address this issue.

6. Radiograph quality – Radiograph quality improvement is crucial in reducing misclassification (over or under-estimation) of lung abnormalities. We found the most common reasons that digital radiographs from Clinic B did not meet Grade 1 criteria for quality were the presence of artifact and exposure problems, which could be readily addressed through ongoing quality control. [NIOSH 2008]. (We provided Clinic B with information on improving quality of digital radiographs [see Appendix B]).

7. ILO classification and awareness among consulting radiologists – We recommend classification of chest radiographs according to the ILO International Classification of Radiographs of Pneumoconioses [ILO 2002]. This classification system allows physicians to describe the degree of dust-related changes present on a chest radiograph and to assess the radiograph quality. ILO standards are now available for digital radiographs (available at: http://www.ilo.org/safework/info/publications/WCMS_168260/lang--en/index.htm). We also recommend increasing the awareness of the concern for interstitial lung diseases among radiologists who assess the surveillance chest radiographs by inserting a comment such as "Rule out indium lung disease/interstitial lung disease/pulmonary alveolar proteinosis" on the request form for the chest radiograph. By being aware of the motivation for these medical surveillance radiographs, hospital-based radiologists will be less likely to miss subtle abnormalities.

8. Referral to pulmonologist – Until more is known about indium-related lung disease, the company should have a low threshold for referring workers to a pulmonologist for additional evaluation. Abnormalities on lung function testing that could indicate early indium-related lung disease (excessive decline in FEV_1, restrictive pattern or obstruction on spirometry, low total lung capacity, and/or low diffusing capacity) should prompt evaluation by a pulmonologist. Such an evaluation would be expected to include repeat testing to confirm the abnormality,

more frequent surveillance (such as every six months) for confirmed abnormalities, and possibly additional diagnostic tests (such as HRCT, more sophisticated lung function tests, and/or bronchoscopy). As noted in the Discussion section of this report, the benefits of frequent, repeated HRCT are probably not warranted by natural history and must be weighed against radiation exposure and cost.

9. Worker reassignment –ITO industry workers with suspected lung disease related to indium compounds should be reassigned to other jobs with minimal exposure. If such reassignment is not possible, then the worker should be provided a PAPR (with assigned protection factor of 1000) and instructed to use that respirator at all times throughout the facility.

Company's Update

In November 2011, the company provided an update to NIOSH on new workplace changes since the September 2010 interim report. Below is a summary of the company's most recent changes.

Engineering Controls

The company is focusing its efforts on those areas with the highest measured levels of dust utilizing a three-pronged approach comprised of these elements: eliminate, segregate, and remediate. They have installed upgraded reclaim milling and mixing equipment. They have segregated the planar grinding process into a separate work space as well as segregating rotary segment cutting. They have purchased two additional enclosed rotary grinding units, an enclosed planar finishing unit, and are in the process of procuring an enclosed planar grinding machine.

Work Practices

The company has developed a comprehensive training program that includes personal protective equipment protocols. They have also instituted an Operator Lead Safety Committee that is responsible for holding monthly meetings and teams of three employees audit all plant areas monthly to assess the environmental health and safety status. Area Supervisors are now responsible for random reviews of safety protocols within their area. A newly hired facility-dedicated EHS manager is responsible for reinforcing

RECOMMENDATIONS
(CONTINUED)

the Respiratory Protection Program, conducting Safety reviews, and mentoring the Safety Committee. In addition, the company has instituted regularly scheduled environmental health and safety updates for all employees.

Industrial Hygiene Testing

The company has verified internal testing results with independent test results obtained from an outside consultant. In 2011, sampling equipment was purchased by the company which will allow for measuring exposure levels throughout the plant including stationary and personal sampling. A full-time facility-dedicated EHS manager was hired in February 2011 and has assumed responsibility for developing a comprehensive testing plan to sample all tasks and jobs a minimum of twice per year.

Medical Surveillance

The company's medical surveillance program includes a physical examination, blood indium level, spirometry, static lung volumes, and diffusing capacity at hire. All production workers and managers spending time in production areas have blood indium level, spirometry, static lung volumes, and diffusing capacity testing annually. Beginning in 2012, surveillance for all production workers and those frequently exposed, including laboratory workers, will be increased to every six months. In addition to screening of all production employees, mandatory yearly screening of all non-production employees will also begin in January 2012.

REFERENCES

American Conference of Governmental Industrial Hygienists (ACGIH) [2001]. Indium and compounds. In: Documentation of the threshold limit values for chemical substances. 7th ed. Cincinnati: ACGIH Worldwide.

Chonan T, Taguchi O, Omae K [2007]. Interstitial pulmonary disorders in indium-processing workers. Eur Respir J 29:317-324.

Collen J, Greenburg D, Holley A, King CS, Hnatiuk O [2008]. Discordance in spirometric interpretations using three commonly used reference equations vs national health and nutrition examination study III. Chest 134:1009-1016.

Collen J, Greenburg D, Holley A, King C, Roop S, Hnatiuk O [2010]. Racial discordance in spirometry comparing four commonly used reference equations to the National Health and Nutrition Examination Study III. Respir Med 104:705-711.

Costabel U, Nakata K [2010]. Pulmonary alveolar proteinosis associated with dust inhalation: not secondary but autoimmune? Am J Respir Crit Care Med 181:427-428.

Cummings KJ, Deubner DC, Day GA, Henneberger PK, Kitt MM, Kent MS, Kreiss K, Schuler CR [2007]. Enhanced preventive program at a beryllium oxide ceramics facility reduces beryllium sensitization among new workers. Occup Environ Med 64:134-140.

Cummings KJ, Donat WE, Ettensohn DB, Roggli VL, Ingram P, Kreiss K [2010a]. Pulmonary alveolar proteinosis in workers at an indium processing facility. Am J Respir Crit Care Med 181:458-464.

Cummings KJ, Kreiss K, Roggli V [2010b]. Pulmonary alveolar proteinosis in workers at an indium processing facility (letter response). Am J Respir Crit Care Med 182:578-579.

Cummings KJ, Nakano M, Omae K, Takeuchi K, Chonan T, Xiao YL, Harley RA, Roggli VL, Hebisawa A, Tallaksen RJ, Trapnell BC, Day GA, Saito R, Stanton ML, Suarthana E, Kreiss K [2011]. Indium lung disease. Chest DOI 10.1378/chest.11-1880.

Department of Health and Human Services (DHHS) [1996]. National Center for Health Statistics. Third National Health and Nutrition Examination Survey, 1988–1994, NHANES III Adult and Examination Data Files (CD-ROM). Public Use Data File Documentation Number 76200. Hyattsville, MD: Centers for Disease Control and Prevention.

Dykstra BJ, Scanlon PD, Kester MM, Beck KC, Enright PL [1999]. Lung volumes in 4,774 patients with obstructive lung disease. Chest 115:68-74.

Gaensler EA, Wright GW [1966]. Evaluation of respiratory impairment. Arch Environ Health 12:146-189.

Goldman HI, Becklake MR [1959]. Respiratory function tests: normal values at median altitudes and the prediction of normal results. Am Rev Tuberc 79: 457-467.

Hamaguchi T, Omae K, Takebayashi T, Kikuchi Y, Yoshioka N, Nishiwaki Y, Tanaka A, Hirata M, Taguchi O, Chonan T [2008]. Exposure to hardly soluble indium compounds in ITO production and recycling plants is a new risk for interstitial lung damage. Occup Environ Med 65:51-55.

Hankinson JL, Odencrantz JR, Fedan KB [1999]. Spirometric reference values from a sample of the general U.S. population. Am J Respir Crit Care Med 159:179-187.

Hnizdo E, Glindmeyer HW, Petsonk EL [2010]. Workplace spirometry monitoring for respiratory disease prevention: a methods review. Int J Tuberc Lung Dis 14:796-805.

Hoet P, De Graef E, Swennen B, Seminck T, Yakoub Y, Deumer G, Haufroid V, Lison D [2011]. Occupational exposure to indium: what does biomonitoring tell us? Toxicol Lett doi:10.1016/j.toxlet.2011.07.004.

Homma T, Ueno T, Sekizawa K, Tanaka A, Hirata M [2003]. Interstitial pneumonia developed in a worker dealing with particles containing indium-tin oxide. J Occup Health 45:137-139.

Homma S, Miyamoto A, Sakamoto S, Kishi K, Motoi N, Yoshimura K [2005]. Pulmonary fibrosis in an individual occupationally exposed to inhaled indium-tin oxide. Eur Respir J 25:200-204.

Inoue Y, Trapnell BC, Tazawa R, Arai T, Takada T, Hizawa N, Kasahara Y, Tatsumi K, Hojo M, Ichiwata T, Tanaka N, Yamaguchi E, Eda R, Oishi K, Tsuchihashi Y, Kaneko C, Nukiwa T, Sakatani M, Krischer JP, Nakata K; Japanese Center of the Rare Lung Diseases Consortium [2008]. Characteristics of a large cohort of patients with autoimmune pulmonary alveolar proteinosis in Japan. Am J Respir Crit Care Med 177:752-762.

International Labour Office (ILO) [2002]. Guidelines for the Use of the ILO International Classification of Radiographs of Pneumoconioses, Revised Edition 2000 (Occupational Safety and Health Series, No. 22). International Labour Office: Geneva.

Ioachimescu OC, Kavuru MS [2006]. Pulmonary alveolar proteinosis. Chron Respir Dis 3:149-159.

Jacobs JH, Meijster T, Meijer E, Suarthana E, Heederik D [2008]. Wheat allergen exposure and the prevalence of work-related sensitization and allergy in bakery workers. Allergy 2008 63:1597-1604.

Klees JE, Ott MG [1999]. Diisocyanates in polyurethane plastics applications. Occup Med 14:759–776.

Knudson RJ, Lebowitz MD, Holberg CJ, Burrows B [1983]. Changes in the normal maximal expiratory flow-volume curve with growth and aging. Am Rev Respir Dis 127:725-734.

Kobayashi J, Kitamura S. KL-6: a serum marker for ILD [1995]. Chest *108*:311-315.

Leach LJ, Scott JK, Armstrong RD, Steadman LT, Maynard EA [1961]. The inhalation toxicity of indium sesquioxide in the rat. Rochester, NY: University of Rochester. Atomic Energy Project Report No. UR-590.

Leroyer C, Perfetti L, Cartier A, Malo JL [1998]. Can reactive airways dysfunction syndrome (RADS) transform into occupational asthma due to "sensitisation" to isocyanates? Thorax *53*:152–153.

Li CY, Sung FC [1999]. A review of the healthy worker effect in occupational epidemiology. Occup Med (Lond) *49*:225–229.

Lison D, Laloy J, Corazzari I, Muller J, Rabolli V, Panin N, Huaux F, Fenoglio I, Fubini B [2009]. Sintered indium-tin-oxide (ITO) particles: a new pneumotoxic entity. Toxicol Sci *108*:472-481.

Lison D, Delos M [2010]. Pulmonary alveolar proteinosis in workers at an indium processing facility. Am J Respir Crit Care Med *15*;182:578.

MacIntyre N, Crapo RO, Viegi G, Johnson DC, van der Grinten CP, Brusasco V, Burgos F, Casaburi R, Coates A, Enright P, Gustafsson P, Hankinson J, Jensen R, McKay R, Miller MR, Navajas D, Pedersen OF, Pellegrino R, Wanger J [2005]. Standardisation of the single-breath determination of carbon monoxide uptake in the lung. Eur Respir J *26*:720-735.

Masuko H, Hizawa N, Chonan T, Amata A, Omae K, Nakano M, Nakata K, Hebisawa A [2011]. Indium-tin oxide does not induce GM-CSF autoantibodies. Am J Respir Crit Care Med *15*;184:741.

Medvedovski E, Alvarez N, Yankov O, Olsson MK [2008]. Advanced indium-tin oxide ceramics for sputtering targets. Ceramics International *34*:1173-1182.

Miller A, Thornton JC, Warshaw R, Anderson H, Teirstein AS, Selikoff IJ [1983]. Single breath diffusing capacity in a representative sample of the population of Michigan, a large industrial state. Predicted values, lower limits of normal, and frequencies of abnormality by smoking history. Am Rev Respir Dis *127*:270-277.

Miller MR, Hankinson J, Brusasco V, Burgos F, Casaburi R, Coates A, Crapo R, Enright P, van der Grinten CP, Gustafsson P, Jensen R, Johnson DC, MacIntyre N, McKay R, Navajas D, Pedersen OF, Pellegrino R, Viegi G, Wanger J; ATS/ERS Task Force [2005]. Standardisation of spirometry. Eur Respir J *26*:319-338.

Ministry of Health, Labor, and Welfare. Technical guidelines for preventing health impairment of workers engaged in the indium tin oxide handling process. Tokyo: Government of Japan; 2010. Available at: http://wwwhourei.mhlw.go.jp/cgi-bin/t_docframe.cgi?MODE=tsuchi&DMODE=CONTENTS&SMODE=NORMAL&KEYWORD=&EFSNO=7276 (in Japanese).

Morris JF, Koski A, Johnson LC [1971]. Spirometric standards for healthy nonsmoking adults. Am Rev Respir Dis 103:57-67.

Nagano K, Gotoh K, Kasai T, Aiso S, Nishizawa T, Ohnishi M, Ikawa N, Eitaki Y, Yamada K, Arito H, Fukushima S [2011]. Two- and 13-week inhalation toxicities of indium-tin oxide and indium oxide in rats. J Occup Health 53:51-63.

Nakano M, Omae K, Tanaka A, Hirata M, Michikawa T, Kikuchi Y, Yoshioka N, Nishiwaki Y, Chonan T [2009]. Causal relationship between indium compound inhalation and effects on the lungs. J Occup Health 51:513-521.

National Institute for Occupational Safety and Health (NIOSH) [2003]. NIOSH Manual of Analytical Methods (NMAM). National Institute for Occupational Safety and Health, Department of Health and Human Services, DHHS (NIOSH) Publication Number 2003-154.

National Institute for Occupational Safety and Health (NIOSH) [2005]. NIOSH Pocket guide to chemical hazards. National Institute for Occupational Safety and Health, Department of Health and Human Services, DHHS (NIOSH) Publication Number 2005-149.

National Institute for Occupational Safety and Health (NIOSH) [2008]. Application of the ILO international classification of radiographs of pneumoconioses to digital chest radiographic images: A NIOSH scientific workshop. National Institute for Occupational Safety and Health, Department of Health and Human Services, DHHS (NIOSH) Publication Number 2008-139.

National Toxicology Program [2001]. Toxicology and carcinogenesis studies of indium phosphide (CAS No. 22398-90-7) in F344/N rats and B6C3F1 mice (inhalation studies). Natl Toxicol Program Tech Rep Ser 499:7-340.

Occupational Safety and Health Administration (OSHA) [2002a]. ID-125G: Metal and Metalloid Particulates in Workplace Atmospheres (Atomic Absorption). Available at: http://www.osha.gov/dts/sltc/methods/inorganic/id121/id121.html.

Occupational Safety and Health Administration (OSHA) [2002b]. ID-125G: Metal and Metalloid Particulates in Workplace Atmospheres (ICP Analysis). Available at: http://www.osha.gov/dts/sltc/methods/inorganic/id125g/id125g.html.

Omae K, Nakano M, Tanaka A, Hirata M, Hamaguchi T, Chonan T [2011]. Indium lung-case reports and epidemiology. Int Arch Occup Environ Health. 84:471-477.

Pellegrino R, Viegi G, Brusasco V, Crapo RO, Burgos F, Casaburi R, Coates A, van der Grinten CP, Gustafsson P, Hankinson J, Jensen R, Johnson DC, MacIntyre N, McKay R, Miller MR, Navajas D,

REFERENCES (CONTINUED)

Pedersen OF, Wanger J [2005]. Interpretative strategies for lung function tests. Eur Respir J 26:948-968.

Ray RL, Salm R [1962]. A fatal case of pulmonary alveolar proteinosis. Thorax 17:257-266.

Seymour JF, Presneill JJ [2002]. Pulmonary alveolar proteinosis: progress in the first 44 years. Am J Respir Crit Care Med 166:215-235.

Smith-Bindman R [2010]. Is computed tomography safe? N Engl J Med 363:1-4.

Sood A, Dawson BK, Henkle JQ, Hopkins-Price P, Quails C [2007]. Effect of change of reference standard to NHANES III on interpretation of spirometric 'abnormality'. Int J Chron Obstruct Pulmon Dis 2:361-367.

State of California [1990]. Test Method 501. Available at: http://www.arb.ca.gov/testmeth/vol1/Meth_501.pdf.

Tanaka A, Hirata M, Omura M, Inoue N, Ueno T, Homma T, Sekizawa K [2002]. Pulmonary toxicity of indium-tin oxide and indium phosphide after intratracheal instillations into the lung of hamsters. J Occup Health 44:99-102.

Tanaka A, Hirata M, Homma T, Kiyohara Y [2010]. Chronic pulmonary toxicity study of indium-tin oxide and indium oxide following intratracheal instillations into the lungs of hamsters. J Occup Health 52:14-22.

Trapnell BC, Whitsett JA, Nakata K [2003]. Pulmonary alveolar proteinosis. N Engl J Med 349:2527-2539.

Wang ML, Avashia BH, Petsonk EL [2006]. Interpreting periodic lung function tests in individuals: the relationship between 1- to 5-year and long-term FEV_1 changes. Chest 130:493-499.

Xiao YL, Cai HR, Wang YH, Meng FQ, Zhang DP [2010]. Pulmonary alveolar proteinosis in an indium-processing worker. Chinese Med J 123:1347-1350.

TABLES

Table 1. Air sampling conducted by the company or its consultants from 2004 to 2010.

Year	Companyor Consultant	Reporting Limit (mcg/sample)	Analyte	Sample Method	Analytical Method
2004	Consultant A	4.0	Indium	Cassette	Modified NIOSH 7300
		± 50	Total Dust	Cassette	NIOSH 0500
2005-2007	Company	0.05	Indium	IOM	OSHA 121/125G
		1.0	Tin Oxide	IOM	OSHA 121/125G
		100	Inhalable Dust	IOM	NIOSH 0500
		100	Respirable Dust	IOM	NIOSH 0600
		1.0	Indium	Cassette	OSHA 121/125G
		1.0	Tin/Tin Oxide	Cassette	OSHA 121/125G
		100	Total Dust	Cassette	NIOSH 0500
		1.0	Indium	Surface Wipe	OSHA 121/125G
		10	(Stages 3, 4, Final, Total Respirable Dust)	Anderson 4-stage Impactor	State of California Method 501
		10	(Stages 1, 2)	Anderson 4-stage Impactor	Gravimetric analysls
2007-2009		1.0	Indium	Cassette	Modified OSHA 125G
		1.0	Tin	Cassette	Modified OSHA 125G
		100	Total Dust	Cassette	Modified NIOSH 0500
2008	Consultant B	0.50	Indium	Cassette	WM001.4.0 in-house
		5.0	Tin	Cassette	WM001.4.0 in-house
		45	Total Weight	Cassette	WM001.01 in-house
2010	Consultant C		Indium	Cassette	NIOSH 7300/ OSHA 125G
			Tin	Cassette	NIOSH 7300/ OSHA 125G
			Total Dust	Cassette	NIOSH 0500

Table 2. Criteria for spirometry grading.

Grade	FVC	FEV$_1$
A	1) $\geq$ 3 acceptable curves* and 2) Best FVC not from last maneuver, or within 50 mL of second best FVC, and 3) FVC repeatable within 100 mL	1) $\geq$ 3 acceptable curves* and 2) Best FEV$_1$ not from last maneuver, or within 50 mL of second best FEV$_1$, and 3) FEV$_1$ repeatable within 100 mL
B	1) $\geq$ 2 acceptable curves* and 2) FVC repeatable within 150 mL	1) $\geq$ 2 acceptable curves* and 2) FEV$_1$ repeatable within 150 mL
C	1) $\geq$ 2 acceptable curves* and 2) FVC repeatable within 250 mL	1) $\geq$ 2 acceptable curves* and 2) FEV$_1$ repeatable within 250 mL
D	Only one acceptable curve*	Only one acceptable curve*
F	No acceptable curves*	No acceptable curves*

*Acceptable curves are those that are free from artifacts, have good starts, and show satisfactory exhalation as per ATS/ERS criteria [Miller et al. 2005].

Table 3. Criteria for excessive decline in FEV$_1$.

Test interval	Lower limit of normal*
< 1.5 years	10.4
1.5 - < 2.5 years	6.1
2.5 - < 3.5 years	4.6
3.5 - < 4.5 years	3.8
$\geq$ 4.5 years	3.2

*Percent change per year [Wang, 2006].

Table 4. Range of surface wipe sampling for indium in 2005 and 2007.

	Surface wipe (N=19)	
Work Area	n	Indium (mcg/cm²)
Administrative	3	3.4 – 4.7
Employee car seats	5	1.5 - 13.7
Men's locker room	2	80 - 101
Lunch room	4	3.0 - 31
ITO sanding - inside respirator mask	1	4
Reclaim - inside respirator mask	1	9.4
Roof - exhaust outlets	3	15 - 109

Table 5. Total and respirable dust, indium, and tin air concentrations measured in four general areas on April 8, 2010.

	Total (mg/m³)			Respirable (mg/m³)		
	Dust	Indium	Tin	Dust	Indium	Tin
Refinery	0.068*	0.018	0.001*	ND†	0.002	0.001†
ITO	0.049*	0.009	0.003	0.058*	0.003	0.002
Grinding	0.091*	0.016	0.001*	ND†	0.002	ND†
Reclaim	0.272	0.136	0.001*	0.135*	0.042	ND†

* < MQC
†ND indicates < MDC

Table 6. Bulk samples collected on April 8, 2010 during the facility visit.

Sample	Description	Department/process	Mass (g)
Indium Hydroxide	White powder	Refinery/filter press	20.03
Indium Oxide	Yellow powder	Refinery	15.13
Tin Oxide	White powder	ITO	12.41
Indium Tin Oxide (ITO)	Yellow liquid-particle suspension (slip)	ITO/casting	71.02
Unsintered ITO	Yellow powder	ITO/sanding room dust collector	54.71
Sintered ITO	Black sintered tiles (small pieces)	ITO/final inspection room	39.01
Sintered ITO	Grey sludge	Grinding/centrifuge	30.69
Sintered and Unsintered ITO	Coarse powder	Reclaim/blender	76.28
Ventilation Dust	Black powder	Reclaim/furnace dust collector #13	19.81
Dross of dross	Dark grey coarse particulate material	Reclaim	34.04
Sludge	Solids in liquid	Refinery/wastewater floor drain	71.60

Table 7. Characteristics of workers participating in the medical surveillance program.

| | Employment Status as of March 18, 2010 | | |
	Current (N=30) n (%)	Former (N=27) n (%)	All (N=57) n (%)
Age at hire (years)			
< 40	15 (50)	18 (67)	33 (58)
≥ 40	15 (50)	9 (33)	24 (42)
Smoking status*			
Ever	22 (73)	13 (48)	35 (61)
Never	5 (17)	1 (4)	6 (11)
Unknown	3 (10)	13 (48)	16 (28)
Body mass index (BMI)†			
Under/normal weight	5 (17)	4 (15)	9 (16)
Overweight	15 (52)	17 (65)	32 (58)
Obese	9 (31)	5 (19)	14 (26)
Tenure (years)‡			
< 4	19 (63)	22 (81)	41 (72)
≥ 4	11 (37)	5 (19)	16 (28)
Surveillance time (months)§			
Mean (range)	38 (0-93)	13 (0-66)	26 (0-93)
Job title category			
Production	22 (73)	20 (74)	42 (74)
ITO grinder	3 (10)	5 (19)	8 (14)
ITO operator	13 (43)	9 (33)	22 (39)
Reclaim operator	3 (10)	4 (15)	7 (12)
Refinery operator	3 (10)	2 (7)	5 (9)
Other	8 (27)	7 (26)	15 (26)
Other with some exposure	5 (17)	4 (15)	9 (16)
Other with minimal exposure	3 (10)	3 (11)	6 (11)

*Determined from spirometry reports. "Ever" includes current and former smokers. "Unknown" refers to workers for whom no smoking information was available.

†Determined from the most recent spirometry reports. BMI ≤ 24.9 kg/m^2 = under/normal weight; 25 – 29.9 kg/m^2 = overweight; ≥ 30 kg/m^2 = obese.

‡Defined as time between hire and 3/18/2010 for current workers and time between hire and termination for former workers.

§Defined as time between first medical surveillance test of any kind and most recent medical surveillance test of any kind. Workers with only one testing interval were assigned a surveillance time of 0 months.

Table 8. Proportions of workers with blood indium level of 5 mcg/L or greater at any time after hire and distributions of the average blood indium level, by work status, hire year, and job category.

Characteristics	Blood indium level ≥5 mcg/L n (%)	Overall median* (range)	Median† for subset with blood indium level ≥5 mcg/L (range)
	N=42	N=42	N=21
All	21 (50)	3.8 (2.5-63)	12 (5.1-63)
Employment Status			
Current	11 (50)	3.8 (2.5-56)	12 (5.1-56)
Former	10 (50)	3.8 (2.5-63)	12 (5.1-63)
Hire year			
< 2007	19 (70)	11.0 (2.5-63)	13 (5.1-63)
≥ 2007	2 (13)	2.5 (2.5-6.2)	5.7 (5.1-6.2)
Job title category			
ITO grinder	4 (57)	5.1 (2.5-56)	24 (5.1-56)
ITO operator	11 (65)	9 (2.5-27)	12 (5.1-27)
Reclaim operator	3 (60)	5.1 (2.5-54)	49 (5.1-54)
Refinery operator	3 (75)	10 (2.5-63)	14 (6.2-63)
Other with some exposure	0 (0)	2.5 (all 2.5)	N/A
Other with minimal exposure	0 (0)	2.5 (all 2.5)	N/A

*Using each worker's most recent after-hire test. Tests with the reported result "none detected" or "0 mcg/L" were assigned a concentration of 2.5 mcg/L, half the reporting value of 5 mcg/L.

†Using each worker's most recent after-hire test. Tests with the reported result "none detected" or "0 mcg/L" were excluded from the analysis.

Table 9a. Quality grades for FVC and FEV$_1$ from 138 spirometry tests on 55 workers.

		FEV1					
		A	B	C	D	F	Total # (%)
FVC	A	12	5	0	0	0	17 (12)
	B	2	26	6	1	0	35 (25)
	C	0	3	0	0	0	3 (2)
	D	0	1	1	21	0	23 (17)
	F	0	0	0	0	60	60 (44)
	Total # (%)	14 (10)	35 (25)	7 (5)	22 (16)	60 (44)	138

Table 9b. Quality grades for FVC and FEV$_1$ from spirometry tests by Clinic A.

		FEV1					
		A	B	C	D	F	Total # (%)
FVC	A	9	3	0	0	0	12 (25)
	B	2	15	4	0	0	21 (45)
	C	0	2	0	0	0	2 (4)
	D	0	1	1	5	0	7 (15)
	F	0	0	0	0	5	5 (11)
	Total # (%)	11 (23)	21 (45)	5 (11)	5 (11)	5 (11)	47

Table 9c. Quality grades for FVC and FEV$_1$ from spirometry tests by Clinic B.

		FEV1					
		A	B	C	D	F	Total # (%)
FVC	A	3	2	0	0	0	5 (6)
	B	0	11	2	1	0	14 (15)
	C	0	1	0	0	0	1 (1)
	D	0	0	0	16	0	16 (18)
	F	0	0	0	0	55	55 (60)
	Total # (%)	3 (3)	14 (15)	2 (2)	17 (19)	55 (60)	91

Table 10. Quality grades for FVC and FEV$_1$ from the most recent spirometry tests of 45 workers tested after hire.

		FEV1					
		A	B	C	D	F	Total # (%)
FVC	A	5	2	0	0	0	7 (16)
	B	0	6	2	0	0	8 (18)
	C	0	1	0	0	0	1 (2)
	D	0	0	0	7	0	7 (16)
	F	0	0	0	0	22	22 (49)
	Total # (%)	5 (11)	9 (20)	2 (4)	7 (16)	22 (49)	45

Table 11. Ever had a restrictive pattern on spirometry after hire, by worker characteristics.

	n (%)
All (N=45)	18 (40)
Employment Status	
Current (N=27)	9 (33)
Former (N=18)	9 (50)
Hire year	
< 2007 (N=25)	13 (52)
≥ 2007 (N=20)	5 (25)
Job title category	
ITO grinder (N=8)	2 (25)
ITO operator (N=17)	8 (47)
Reclaim operator (N=5)	2 (40)
Refinery operator (N=4)	1 (25)
Other with some exposure (N=7)	4 (57)
Other with minimal exposure (N=4)	1 (25)
Blood indium (available in N=39)	
≥ 5 mcg/L (N=20)	9 (45)
< 5 mcg/L (N=19)	6 (32)

Table 12. Comparison of restrictive pattern on the most recent after-hire spirometry test to U.S. adult population (NHANES III) data.*

	N	Observed number	Expected number	Prevalence ratio (95% CI)†
Overall	43	14	3.5	4.0 (2.4-6.7)
Employment status				
Current workers	25	7	2.2	3.2 (1.5-6.5)
Former workers	18	7	1.3	5.4 (2.6-11.0)
Hire year				
< 2007	24	9	1.7	5.3 (2.8-10.1)
≥ 2007	19	5	1.8	2.8 (1.2-6.4)
Job title category				
ITO operator	15	5	1.1	4.6 (2.0-10.7)
ITO grinder	8	2	0.6	3.3 (0.9-12.0)
Other – some exposure	7	4	0.8	5.2 (2.0-13.5)

*NHANES comparison was done in 43 workers. Two workers were Asian and not included in the analysis because expected values for this race were not available. Includes all quality tests.

†Reflects ratio of observed prevalence to expected prevalence and was determined using indirect standardization for race, sex, age, cigarette smoking status, and body mass index. Workers for whom smoking status was unavailable were assumed to be smokers. CI=confidence interval.

Table 13. Comparison of at-hire and most recent spirometry interpretations for 18 workers tested at hire and during employment.*

	Most recent interpretation		
	NORMAL	OBSTRUCTION	RESTRICTIVE
At-hire interpretation			
NORMAL	9	1†	3‡
OBSTRUCTION	0	1	0
RESTRICTIVE	1	0	3

*None of the 18 workers included in this analysis had a mixed pattern.

†One had excessive decline in FEV_1

‡Three had excessive decline in FEV_1

TABLES (CONTINUED)

Table 14a. Ever had an excessive decline in FEV_1 after hire, by worker characteristics.*

	n (%)
Total (N=41)	12 (29)
Employment Status	
Current (N=27)	8 (30)
Former (N=14)	4 (29)
Hire year	
< 2007 (N=22)	8 (36)
≥ 2007 (N=19)	4 (21)
Job title category	
ITO Grinder (N=7)	4 (57)
ITO Operator (N=15)	5 (33)
Reclaim Operator (N=5)	1 (20)
Refinery Operator (N=4)	0 (0)
Other with some exposure (N=7)	1 (14)
Other with minimal exposure (N=3)	1 (33)
Blood indium (available in N=35)	
≥ 5 mcg/L (N=19)	7 (37)
< 5 mcg/L (N=16)	3 (19)

*Five workers with spirometry interpretation of obstruction were included in these analyses.

Table 14b. Ever had an excessive decline in FEV_1 after hire,
by worker characteristics.*

	n (%)
Total (N=36)	8 (22)
Employment Status	
Current (N=22)	4 (18)
Former (N=14)	4 (29)
Hire year	
< 2007 (N=19)	5 (26)
≥ 2007 (N=17)	3 (18)
Job title category	
ITO grinder (N=5)	2 (40)
ITO operator (N=12)	3 (25)
Reclaim operator (N=5)	1 (20)
Refinery operator (N=4)	0 (0)
Other with some exposure (N=7)	1 (14)
Other with minimal exposure (N=3)	1 (33)
Blood indium (available in N=31)	
≥ 5 mcg/L (N=16)	4 (25)
< 5 mcg/L (N=15)	3 (20)

*Five workers with spirometry interpretation of obstruction were excluded from these analyses.

Table 15. Ever had low total lung capacity (TLC) after hire, by worker characteristics.

	n (%)
Total (N=35)	8 (23)
Employment Status	
Current (N=27)	7 (26)
Former (N=8)	1 (13)
Hire year	
< 2007 (N=15)	5 (33)
≥ 2007 (N=20)	3 (13)
Job title category	
ITO grinder (N=6)	0 (0)
ITO operator (N=12)	3 (25)
Reclaim operator (N=5)	2 (40)
Refinery operator (N=3)	0 (0)
Other with some exposure (N=6)	3 (50)
Other with minimal exposure (N=3)	0 (0)
Blood indium (available in N=29)	
≥ 5 mcg/L (N=14)	4 (29)
< 5 mcg/L (N=15)	2 (13)

Table 16. Ever had low diffusing capacity (DLCO) after hire, by worker characteristics.

	n (%)
Total (N=35)	8 (23)
Employment Status	
Current (N=27)	5 (19)
Former (N=8)	3 (38)
Hire year	
< 2007 (N=15)	4 (27)
≥ 2007 (N=20)	4 (25)
Job title category	
ITO grinder (N=6)	2 (33)
ITO operator (N=12)	4 (33)
Reclaim operator (N=5)	1 (20)
Refinery operator (N=3)	0 (0)
Other with some exposure (N=6)	1 (17)
Other with minimal exposure (N=3)	0 (0)
Blood indium (available in N=29)	
≥ 5 mcg/L (N=14)	4 (29)
< 5 mcg/L (N=15)	4 (27)

Table 17a. Agreement between restrictive pattern on spirometry and excessive decline in FEV_1.*

		Restrictive pattern		Total
		No	Yes	
Excessive decline	No	20	9	29
	Yes	5	7	12
Total		25	16	41

*Five workers with spirometry interpretation of obstruction were included in these analyses.

Table 17b. Agreement between restrictive pattern on spirometry and excessive decline in FEV_1.*

		Restrictive pattern		Total
		No	Yes	
Excessive decline	No	19	9	28
	Yes	1	7	8
Total		20	16	36

*Five workers with spirometry interpretation of obstruction were excluded from these analyses.

Table 17c. Agreement between restrictive pattern on spirometry and low total lung capacity (TLC).

		Restrictive pattern		Total
		No	Yes	
TLC	Normal	22	5	27
	Low	1	7	8
Total		23	12	35

Table 17d. Agreement between restrictive pattern on spirometry and low diffusing capacity (DLCO).

		Restrictive pattern		Total
		No	Yes	
DLCO	Normal	18	9	27
	Low	5	3	8
Total		23	12	35

Table 17e. Agreement between low total lung capacity (TLC) and low diffusing capacity (DLCO).

		TLC		Total
		Normal	Low	
DLCO	Normal	21	6	27
	Low	6	2	8
Total		27	8	35

Table 18. Summary of exposure estimates and adverse health outcomes ever after hire by job title category.

	ITO Grinder	ITO Operator	Reclaim Operator	Refinery Operator	Other jobs some exposure	Other jobs minimal exposure
Indium exposure (mg/m³)*	0.17 (0.1 - 0.5) n = 8	0.13 (0.03 - 0.6) n = 15	0.7 (0.06 - 4.0) n = 10	1.5 (0.5 - 3.6) n = 5	N/A	N/A
Blood indium level ≥ 5 mcg/L	57% (4/7)	65% (11/17)	60% (3/5)	75% (3/4)	0 (0/5)	0 (0/4)
Restrictive pattern on spirometry	25% (2/8)	47% (8/17)	40% (2/5)	25% (1/4)	57% (4/7)	25% (1/4)
Excessive decline FEV_1	57% (4/7)	33% (5/15)	20% (1/5)	0 (0/4)	14% (1/7)	33% (1/3)
Restriction (low total lung capacity)	0 (0/6)	25% (3/12)	40% (2/5)	0 (0/3)	50% (3/6)	0 (0/3)
Low diffusing capacity	33% (2/6)	33% (4/12)	20% (1/5)	0 (0/3)	17% (1/6)	0 (0/3)
Abnormal CXR†	0 (0/3)	0% (0/13)	67% (2/3)	0 (0/3)	0 (0/5)	0 (0/1)
Case of pulmonary alveolar proteinosis	0 (0/8)	5% (1/22)	0 (0/7)‡	0 (0/5)	0 (0/9)	0 (0/5)

*GM (range) for full- or partial-shift historical personal samples analyzed for total indium

†In addition, two former workers (one reclaim operator, one ITO operator) had diffuse abnormalities on chest radiographs done after hire outside of the formal surveillance program.

‡One case occurred in a Reclaim Operator prior to the company's purchase of the facility.

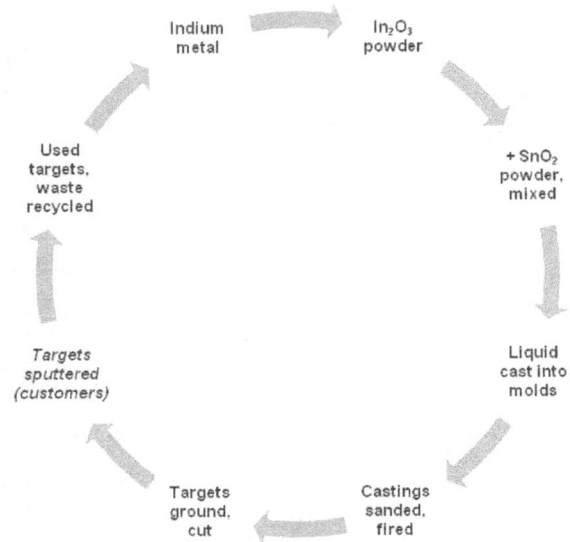

Figure 1. Production of indium-tin oxide targets and reclamation of indium metal.

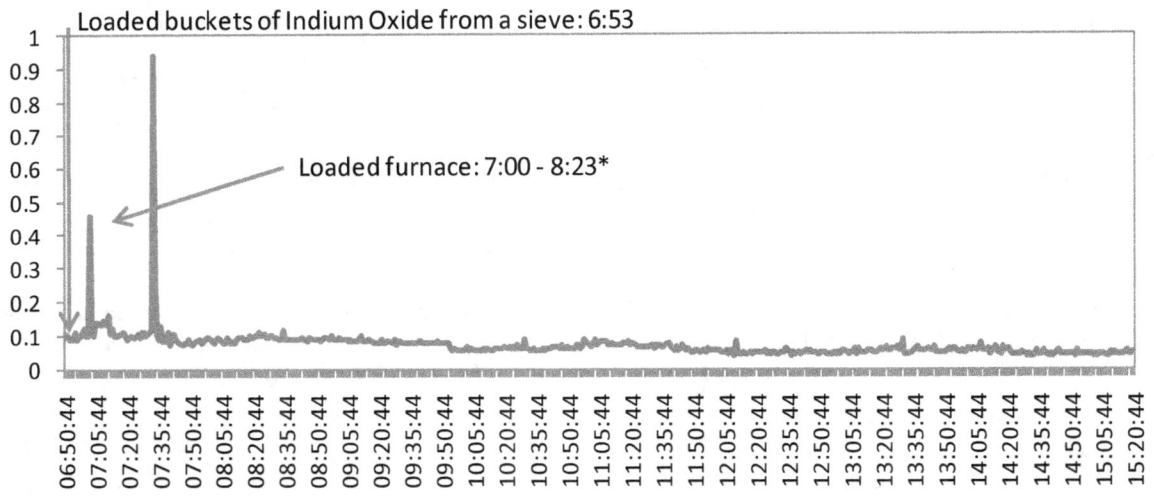

Figure 2. Real-time air dust concentrations in the refinery area on April 8, 2010. The average concentration over 513 minutes sampling period was 0.07 mg/m³. *The task was completed sometime between 7:00 and 8:23.

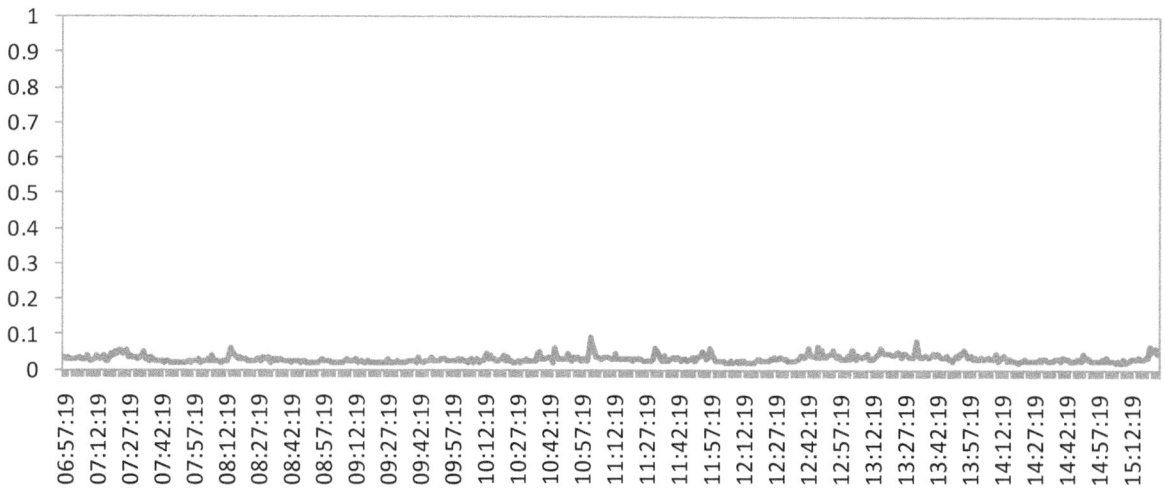

Figure 3. Real-time air dust concentrations in the ITO department on April 8, 2010. The average concentration over 509 minutes sampling period was 0.031 mg/m³.

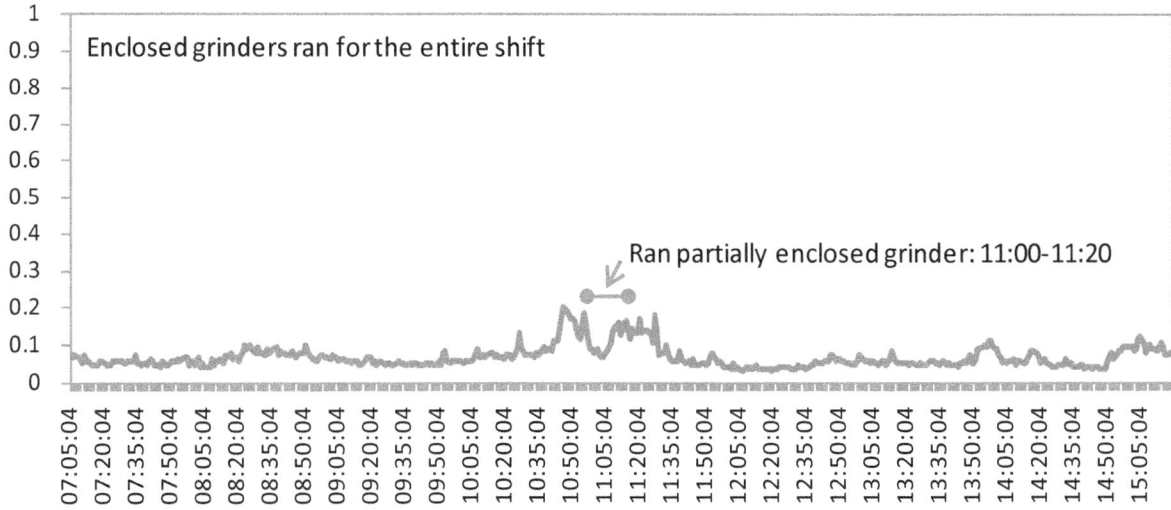

Figure 4. Real-time air dust concentrations in the grinding area on April 8, 2010. The average concentration over 496 minutes sampling period was 0.068 mg/m³.

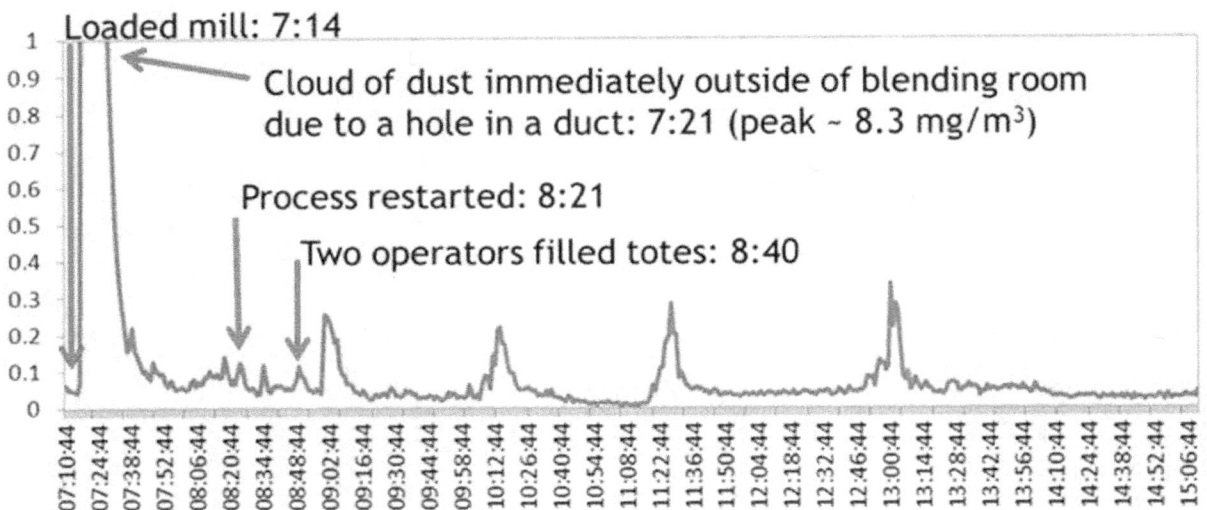

Figure 5. Real-time air dust concentrations in the reclaim area on April 8, 2010. The average concentration over 478 minutes sampling period was 0.168 mg/m³. Four peaks of approximately 0.25 mg/m³ were observed between 8:50 and 13:14 (no task identification due to the lack of observation).

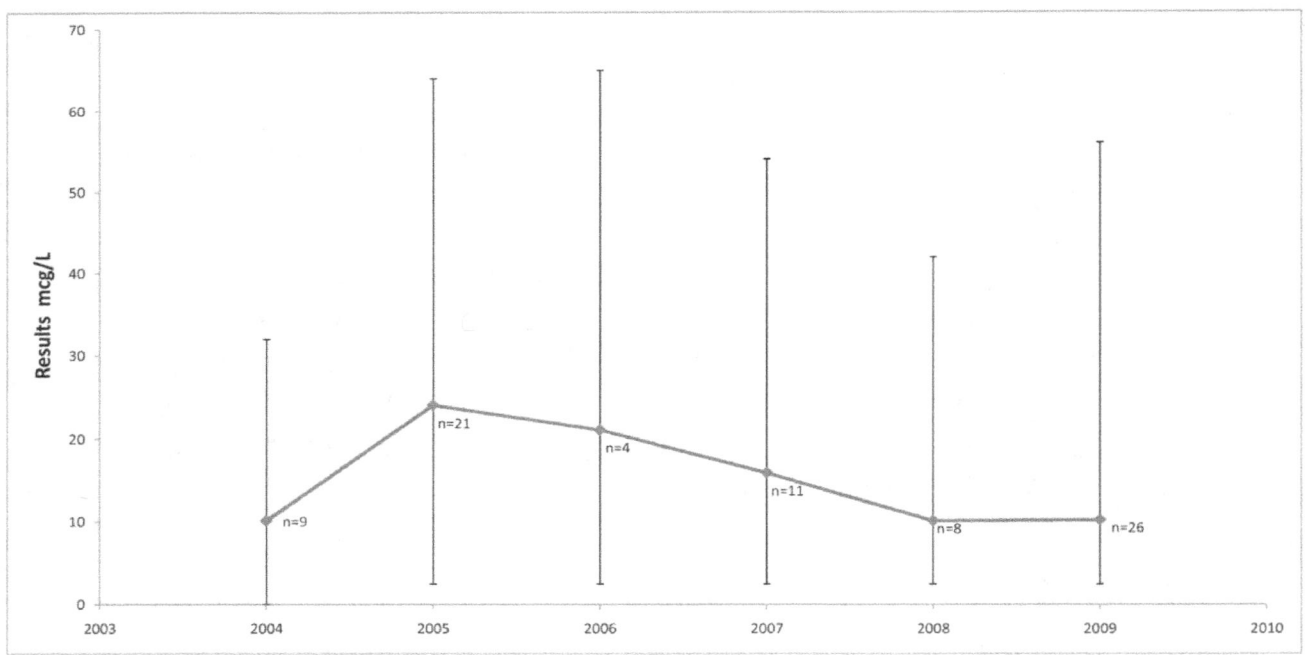

Figure 6. Mean and range of after-hire blood indium level by year. Tests with the reported result "none detected" were assigned a concentration of 2.5 mcg/L, half the reporting value of 5 mcg/L.

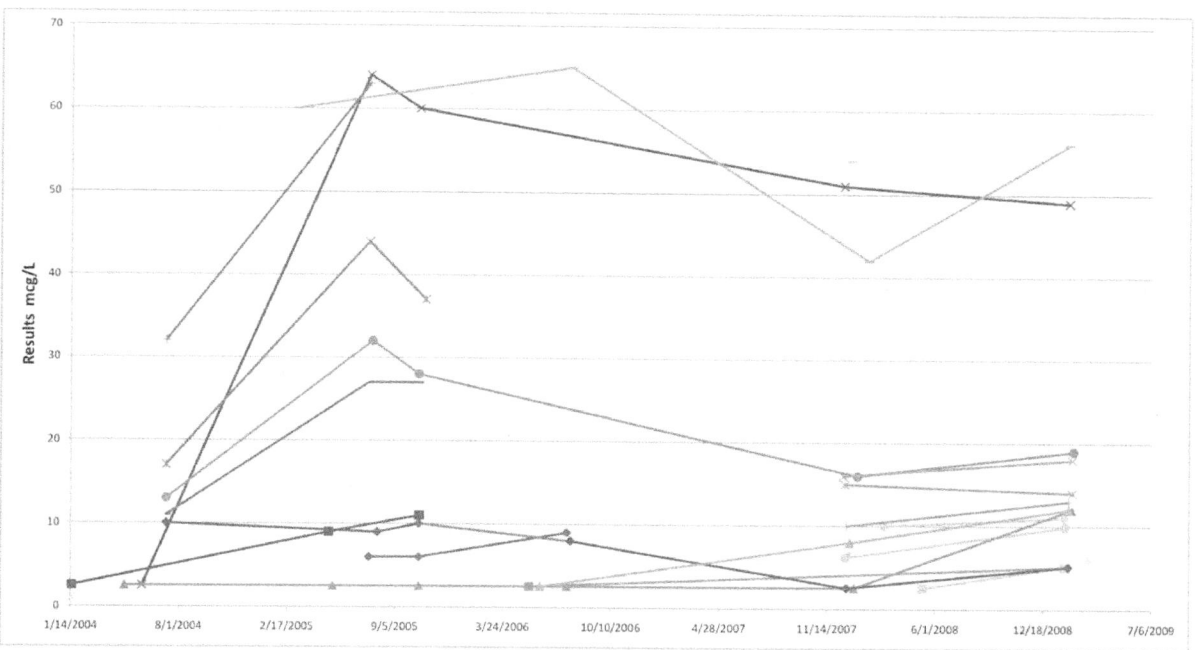

Figure 7. Blood indium level over time for 21 workers with blood indium concentration of 5 mcg/L or greater at any time after hire. Tests done at hire are included, if available.

A.1. Number of samples

Number of Personal Air Samples by Sample Type

	Number of Personal Partial- to Full-Shift / Short Duration by Sample Type		
	Cassette	IOM	Cyclone
Total Dust	37/25	---	2/0
Total Indium	38/25	---	4/1
Total Tin	30/12	---	---
Inhalable Dust	--- *	9/4	---
Inhalable Indium	---	2/1	---
Inhalable Tin	---	0/0	---
Respirable Dust	---	9/4	---
Respirable Indium	---	9/4	---
Respirable Tin	---	8/3	---

* Sample not collected

Number of General Area Air Samples by Sample Type

	Number of Area Partial- to Full-Shift / Short Duration by Sample Type	
	Cassette	IOM
Total Dust	21/4	---
Total Indium	21/4	---
Total Tin	9/1	---
Inhalable Dust	---*	0/1
Inhalable Indium	---	---
Inhalable Tin	---	---
Respirable Dust	---	0/1
Respirable Indium	---	0/1
Respirable Tin	---	0/0

* Sample not collected

Number of Personal IOM Samples by Work Area

Work Area	Dust Inhalable Partial- to Full-Shift	Dust Inhalable Short Duration	Dust Respirable Partial- to Full-Shift	Dust Respirable Short Duration	Indium Inhalable Partial- to Full-Shift	Indium Inhalable Short Duration	Indium Respirable Partial- to Full-Shift	Indium Respirable Short Duration	Tin Inhalable Partial- to Full-Shift	Tin Inhalable Short Duration	Tin Respirable Partial- to Full-Shift	Tin Respirable Short Duration
ITO Department	3	--*	3	--	--	1	3	2	--	--	3	--
Grinding	4	2	4	2	1	--	4	--	--	--	3	1
Reclaim	2	--	2	--	1	--	2	--	--	--	2	--
Refinery	--	2	--	2	--	--	--	2	--	--	--	2
Total	9	4	9	4	2	1	9	4	--	--	8	3

* Sample not collected

Number of Personal Cassettes by Work Area for Indium (In) and Tin (Sn) by Year – Partial- to Full-Shift Duration

Work Area	2004 In	2004 Sn	2005 In	2005 Sn	2006 In	2006 Sn	2007 In	2007 Sn	2008 In	2008 Sn	2009 In	2009 Sn	2010 In	2010 Sn	Total In	Total Sn
ITO Dept	--*	--	--	--	1	1	5	2	5	5	3	3	1	1	15	12
Grinding	--	--	--	--	--	--	3	2	1	1	4	4	--	--	8	7
Reclaim	--	--	--	--	--	--	3	1	3	3	2	2	2	2	10	8
Refinery	--	--	--	--	--	--	3	1	1	1	1	1	--	--	5	3
Total					1	1	14	6	10	10	10	10	3	3	38	30

* Sample not collected

Number of Personal Cassettes by Work Area for Indium (In) and Tin (Sn) by Year – Short Duration

Work Area	2004 In	2004 Sn	2005 In	2005 Sn	2006 In	2006 Sn	2007 In	2007 Sn	2008 In	2008 Sn	2009 In	2009 Sn	2010 In	2010 Sn	Total In	Total Sn
ITO Dept	---*	---	---	---	---	---	3	3	---	---	---	---	---	---	3	3
Grinding	---	---	---	---	1	1	2	2	---	---	---	---	---	---	3	3
Reclaim	---	---	---	---	---	---	---	---	1	1	---	---	---	---	1	1
Refinery	9	---	---	---	2	2	6	2	1	1	---	---	---	---	18	5
Total	9	---	---	---	3	3	11	7	2	2	---	---	---	---	25	12

* Sample not collected

A.2. Concentrations

A.2.1 Concentrations (in mg/m³) by Work Area by Sample Duration in Personal Air Cassette Samples

Personal Cassette Indium (N=63)

Work Area	n	Partial- to Full-Shift Range	Partial- to Full-Shift Mean	Partial- to Full-Shift Geometric Mean	n	Short Duration Range	Short Duration Mean	Short Duration Geometric Mean
ITO department	15	0.03 – 0.59	0.18	0.13	3	0.07 – 0.45	0.31	0.23
Grinding	8	0.07 – 0.45	0.19	0.17	3	0.17 – 0.26	0.23	0.22
Reclaim	10	0.06 – 4.0	1.3	0.74	1		0.10	0.10
Refinery	5	0.47 – 3.6	1.8	1.5	18	0.03 – 46	6.6	1.9
Total	38				25			

Personal Cassette Tin (N=42)

Work Area	n	Partial- to Full-Shift Range	Partial- to Full-Shift Mean	Partial- to Full-Shift Geometric Mean	n	Short Duration Range	Short Duration Mean	Short Duration Geometric Mean
ITO department	12	0.0005 – 0.03	0.006	0.003	3	0.0015 – 0.002	0.002	0.002
Grinding	7	0.005 – 0.02	0.01	0.01	3	0.01 – 0.03	0.02	0.02
Reclaim	8	0.002 – 0.12	0.04	0.02	1		0.01	0.01
Refinery	3	0.001 – 0.003	0.002	0.001	5	0.002 – 0.08	0.02	0.006
Total	30				12			

Personal Cassette Total Dust (N=62)

Work Area	n	Partial- to Full-Shift Range	Partial- to Full-Shift Mean	Partial- to Full-Shift Geometric Mean	n	Short Duration Range	Short Duration Mean	Short Duration Geometric Mean
ITO department	15	0.05 – 0.89	0.32	0.24	3	0.16 – 0.93	0.65	0.50
Grinding	8	0.20 – 0.85	0.40	0.36	3	0.49 – 1.10	0.75	0.71
Reclaim	10	0.22 – 5.2	2.0	1.2	1		0.13	0.13
Refinery	4	0.68 – 6.4	3.0	2.1	18	0.35 – 65.0	10.0	3.2
Total	37				25			

Personal Cyclone Indium (N=5)

Work Area	n	Partial- to Full-Shift Range	Partial- to Full-Shift Mean	Partial- to Full-Shift Geometric Mean	n	Short Duration Range	Short Duration Mean	Short Duration Geometric Mean
Grinding	3	0.0004 – 0.11	0.04	0.01	---			
ITO Dept	---*				1		0.03	0.03
Reclaim	1		0.27	0.27	---			
Total	4				1			

*Sample not collected

Personal Cyclone Total Dust (N=2)

	n	Partial- to Full-Shift Range	Partial- to Full-Shift Mean	Partial- to Full-Shift GM	n	Short Duration Range	Short Duration Mean	Short Duration GM
Grinding	2	0.217 – 0.218	0.22	0.22	---*			

* Sample not collected

A.2.2. Concentrations (in mg/m³) by Work Area by Year in Personal Air Cassette Samples

Geometric Mean Indium Concentrations by Work Area by Year in Personal Cassette Samples – Partial- to Full-Shift Duration

Work Area	2004	2005	2006	2007	2008	2009	2010
ITO Dept	--*	---	0.25 n=1	0.13 n=5	0.15 n=5	0.10 n=3	0.07 n=1
Grinding	---	---	---	0.19 n=3	0.17 n=1	0.15 n=4	---
Reclaim	---	---	---	1.4 n=3	0.53 n=3	3.3 n=2	0.10 n=2
Refinery	---	---	---	1.2 n=3	1.1 n=1	3.6 n=1	---

* No sample collected

Geometric Mean Indium Concentrations by Work Area by Year in Personal Cassette Samples – Short Duration

Work Area	2004	2005	2006	2007	2008	2009	2010
ITO Dept	--*	---	---	0.23 n=3	---	---	---
Grinding	---	---	0.16 n=1	0.26 n=2	---	---	---
Reclaim	---	---	---	---	0.10 n=1	---	---
Refinery	3.3 n=9	---	3.4 n=2	0.9 n=6	0.5 n=1	---	---

* No sample collected

Geometric Mean Total Dust Concentrations by Work Area by Year in Personal Cassette Samples – Partial- to Full-Shift Duration

Work Area	2004	2005	2006	2007	2008	2009	2010
ITO Dept	--*	---	0.57 n=1	0.26 n=5	0.27 n=5	0.13 n=3	0.22 n=1
Grinding	---	---	---	0.51 n=3	0.25 n=1	0.31 n=4	---
Reclaim	---	---	---	2.6 n=3	0.67 n=3	3.9 n=2	0.33 n=2
Refinery	---	---	---	2.6 n=3	1.1 n=1	---	---

* No sample collected

Geometric Mean Total Dust Concentrations by Work Area by Year in Personal Cassette Samples – Short Duration

Work Area	2004	2005	2006	2007	2008	2009	2010
ITO Dept	--*	---	---	0.50 n=3	---	---	---
Grinding	---	---	0.68 n=1	0.73 n=2	---	---	---
Reclaim	---	---	---	---	0.13 n=1	---	---
Refinery	4.3 n=9	---	4.8 n=2	2.4 n=6	0.53 n=1	---	---

* No sample collected

A.2.3. Concentrations (in mg/m³) by Work Area by Sample Duration in General Area Cassette Samples

Area Cassette Indium (N=25)

Work Area	n	Partial- to Full-Shift Range	Partial- to Full-Shift Mean	Partial- to Full-Shift Geometric Mean	n	Short Duration Range	Short Duration Mean	Short Duration Geometric Mean
Grinding	13	0.002 – 0.45	0.08	0.03	3	0.01 – 0.07	0.04	0.03
ITO Department	3	0.009 – 0.02	0.01	0.01	1		0.17	0.17
Reclaim	5	0.02 – 4.5	1.4	0.45	---*			
Total	21				4			

* No sample collected

Area Cassette Tin (N=10)

Work Area	n	Partial- to Full-Shift Range	Partial- to Full-Shift Mean	Partial- to Full-Shift Geometric Mean	n	Short Duration Range	Short Duration Mean	Short Duration Geometric Mean
Grinding	2	0.007 – 0.02	0.01	0.01	1		.01	.01
ITO Department	3	0.0009 – 0.001	0.001	0.001	---*			
Reclaim	4	0.001 – 0.37	0.11	0.02	---			
Total	9				1			

* No sample collected

Area Cassette Total Dust (N=25)

Work Area	n	Partial- to Full-Shift Range	Partial- to Full-Shift Mean	Partial- to Full-Shift GM	n	Partial- to Full-Shift Range	Partial- to Full-Shift Mean	Partial- to Full-Shift GM
Grinding	13	0.05 – 0.85	0.27	0.20	3	0.25 – 1.0	0.61	0.52
ITO Department	3	0.02 – 0.14	0.06	0.04	1		0.63	0.63
Reclaim	5	0.16 – 6.6	2.3	1.2	---*			
Total	21				4			

* No sample collected

A.2.4. Concentrations (in mg/m³) by department by year in general area cassette samples

Geometric Mean Indium Concentrations by Work Area by Year in General Area Cassette Samples – Partial- to Full-Shift Duration

Work Area	2004	2005	2006	2007	2008	2009	2010
ITO Dept	---*	0.01 n=3	---	---	---	---	---
Grinding	---	0.03 n=13	---	---	---	---	---
Reclaim	---	1.0 n=2	4.5 n=1	---	---	---	0.06 n=2
Refinery	---	---	---	---	---	---	---

* No sample collected

Geometric Mean Indium Concentrations by Work Area by Year in General Area Cassette Samples – Short Duration

Work Area	2004	2005	2006	2007	2008	2009	2010
ITO Dept	---*	0.17 n=1	---	---	---	---	---
Grinding	---	0.03 n=3	---	---	---	---	---
Reclaim	---		---	---	---	---	---
Refinery	---		---	---	---	---	---

* No sample collected

Geometric Mean Total Dust Concentrations by Work Area by Year in General Area Cassette Samples – Partial- to Full-Shift Duration

Work Area	2004	2005	2006	2007	2008	2009	2010
ITO Dept	---*	.04 n=3	---	---	---	---	---
Grinding	---	0.20 n=13	---	---	---	---	---
Reclaim	---	2.1 n=2	6.6 n=1	---	---	---	0.28 n=2
Refinery	---	---	---	---	---	---	---

* No sample collected

Geometric Mean Total Dust Concentrations by Work Area by Year in General Area Cassette Samples – Short Duration

Work Area	2004	2005	2006	2007	2008	2009	2010
ITO Dept	---*	.63 n=1	---	---	---	---	---
Grinding	---	---	0.52 n=3	---	---	---	---
Reclaim	---	---	---	---	---	---	---
Refinery	---	---	---	---	---	---	---

* No sample collected

A.2.5. Concentrations (in mg/m³) by Work Area by Size and Duration in Personal IOM Samples

Personal IOM Indium (N=11)
Partial- to Full-Shift

Work Area	Inhalable n	Inhalable Range	Inhalable Mean	Inhalable Geometric Mean	Respirable n	Respirable Range	Respirable Mean	Respirable Geometric Mean
Grinding	1		0.41	0.41	4	0.01 – 0.03	0.02	0.02
ITO Department	--*				3	0.03 – 0.08	0.06	0.05
Reclaim	1		3.3	3.3	2	0.11 – 1.1	0.62	0.35
Total	2				9			

* No sample collected

Personal IOM Indium (N=5)
Short Duration

Work Area	Inhalable n	Inhalable Range	Inhalable Mean	Inhalable Geometric Mean	Respirable n	Respirable Range	Respirable Mean	Respirable Geometric Mean
Grinding	--*				2	0.01 – 0.04	0.02	0.02
ITO Department	1		0.62	0.62	---			
Reclaim	---				---			
Refinery	---				2	0.21 – 0.47	0.34	0.31
Total	1				4			

* No sample collected

Personal IOM Tin (N=8)
Partial-- to Full--Shift

Work Area	Inhalable n	Inhalable Range	Inhalable Mean	Inhalable Geometric Mean	Respirable n	Respirable Range	Respirable Mean	Respirable Geometric Mean
Grinding	---*				3	0.001 – 0.002	0.002	0.001
ITO Department	---				3	0.001 – 0.004	0.002	0.001
Reclaim	---				2	0.09 – 0.89	0.49	0.28
Total	0				8			

* No sample collected

Personal IOM Tin (N=3)
Short Duration

Work Area	Inhalable n	Inhalable Range	Inhalable Mean	Inhalable Geometric Mean	Respirable n	Respirable Range	Respirable Mean	Respirable Geometric Mean
Grinding	---*				1		0.002	0.002
Refinery	---				2	0.003 – 0.005	0.004	0.004
Total	0				3			

*No sample collected

Personal IOM Total Dust (N=9)
Partial- to Full-Shift

Work Area	Inhalable n	Inhalable Range	Inhalable Mean	Inhalable Geometric Mean	Respirable n	Respirable Range	Respirable Mean	Respirable Geometric Mean
Grinding	4	0.05 – 1.1	0.44	0.26	4	0.05 – 0.21	0.15	0.13
ITO Department	3	0.37 – 1.6	0.79	0.63	3	0.18 – 0.27	0.21	0.21
Reclaim	2	3.8 – 14	8.7	7.2	2	0.56 – 2.1	1.3	1.1
Total	9				9			

Personal IOM Total Dust (N=4)
Short Duration

Work Area	Inhalable n	Inhalable Range	Inhalable Mean	Inhalable Geometric Mean	Respirable n	Respirable Range	Respirable Mean	Respirable Geometric Mean
Grinding	2	1.01 – 1.04	1.0	1.0	2	0.71 – 1.04	0.88	0.86
ITO Department	---*				---			
Reclaim	---				---			
Refinery	2	7.1 – 8.9	8.0	8.0	2	2.0 – 2.1	2.0	2.0
Total	4				4			

* No sample collected

A.2.6. Concentrations (in mg/m³) by Work Area by Size in Area IOM samples

Area IOM Indium (N=1) Short Duration

Work Area	Inhalable n	Inhalable Range	Inhalable Mean	Inhalable Geometric Mean	Respirable n	Respirable Range	Respirable Mean	Respirable Geometric Mean
Grinding	--*				1		0.03	0.03

*No sample collected

Area IOM Total Dust (N=1) Short Duration

Work Area	Inhalable n	Inhalable Range	Inhalable Mean	Inhalable Geometric Mean	Respirable n	Respirable Range	Respirable Mean	Respirable Geometric Mean
Grinding	1		.25	0.25	1		0.25	0.25

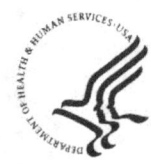

DEPARTMENT OF HEALTH & HUMAN SERVICES

Phone: (304) 285-5751
Fax: (304) 285-5820

Public Health Service

Centers for Disease Control
and Prevention (CDC)
National Institute for Occupational
Safety and Health (NIOSH)
1095 Willowdale Road
Morgantown, WV 26505-2888

April 16, 2010

Physician
Clinic B

Dear Doctor,

On behalf of the NIOSH team that visited the indium-tin oxide production facility in Rhode Island from April 7-9, 2010, we would like to thank you for taking the time to meet with us. As part of our Health Hazard Evaluation, we arranged for the digitally-acquired chest radiographs from your institution to be classified according to the ILO Classification System by two or more NIOSH B readers.

The ILO Classification System includes an assessment of radiograph quality as follows:

Grade 1: Good
Free of technical imperfections or artifacts

Grade 2: Acceptable
No technical defects or artifacts likely to impair classification

Grade 3: Acceptable
With technical defects or artifacts but still adequate for classification

Grade 4: U/R
Unacceptable for classification

If quality is not Grade 1, an indication of the technical defect(s) is made. Minor errors in positioning and handling artifacts that do not overlie the heart or lungs would usually be classified as Grade 2; minor degrees of over- or underexposure and minor departures from proper radiographic contrast would usually be classified as Grade 3; and gross over- or underexposure, gross unsharpness due to motion or poor contact, and gross departures from proper radiographic contrast as U/R.

During our visit, we provided some feedback on the quality of the digitally-acquired radiographs from your institution. None of the radiographs we reviewed had Grade 1 quality and many had Grade 3 quality. The B readers indicated that the radiographs had problems with mottle (which refers to grainy, blotchy, textured, or snowy appearance in a radiographic image) and exposure. Such quality issues can lead to misclassification of radiographs. Defects can be misinterpreted to represent disease when none exists, or true interstitial lung disease can be misinterpreted as radiographic artifact. Either form of misclassification would impact your efforts to conduct medical surveillance.

Enclosed you will find a list of the radiographs reviewed and the B reader's classification, including

quality grading. We hope this information and the CD we provided containing NIOSH Publication No. 2008-139 (Application of the ILO International Classification of Radiographs of Pneumoconioses to Digital Chest Radiographic Images, A NIOSH Scientific Workshop) are helpful to you and the radiology department. Please do not hesitate to contact us if additional questions arise.

Sincerely,

Kristin Cummings, MD, MPH

Eva Suarthana, MD, PhD
Field Studies Branch
Division of Respiratory Disease Studies

Acknowledgements and Availability of Report

The Respiratory Disease Hazard Evaluation and Technical Assistance Program of NIOSH conducts field investigations of possible health hazards in the workplace. These investigations are conducted under the authority of Section 20(a)(6) of the Occupational Safety and Health (OSH) Act of 1970, 29 U.S.C. 669(a)(6), or Section 501(a)(11) of the Federal Mine Safety and Health Act of 1977, 30 U.S.C. 951(a)(11), which authorizes the Secretary of Health and Human Services, following a written request from any employers or authorized representative of employees, to determine whether any substance normally found in the place of employment has potentially toxic effects in such concentrations as used or found.

The Respiratory Disease Hazard Evaluation and Technical Assistance Program also provides, upon request, technical and consultative assistance to federal, state, and local agencies; labor; industry; and other groups or individuals to control occupational health hazards and to prevent related trauma and disease.

Mention of any company or product does not constitute endorsement by NIOSH. In addition, citations to websites external to NIOSH do not constitute NIOSH endorsement of the sponsoring organizations or their programs or products. Furthermore, NIOSH is not responsible for the content of these websites. All Web addresses referenced in this document were accessible as of the publication date.

This report was prepared by Kristin Cummings, Eva Suarthana, Gregory A. Day, Marcia L. Stanton, Rena Saito, and Kathleen Kreiss, of the Field Studies Branch, Division of Respiratory Disease Studies. Analytical support was provided by Nicole Edwards and Xiaoming Liang. Statistical support was provided by Kathy Fedan. Desktop publishing was performed by Tia McClelland.

Copies of this report have been sent to employee and management representatives at the requesting company, the state health department, and the OSHA Regional Office. This report is not copyrighted and may be freely reproduced. The report may be viewed and printed at www.cdc.gov/niosh/hhe/. Copies may be purchased from the National Technical Information Service (NTIS) at 5825 Port Royal Road, Springfield, Virginia 22161.

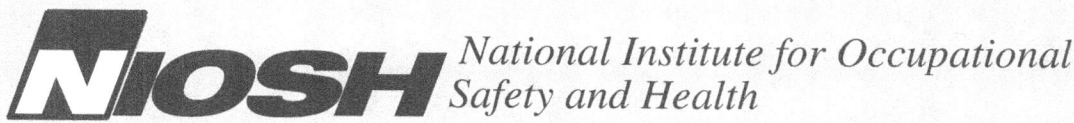

National Institute for Occupational Safety and Health

Delivering on the Nation's promise: Safety and health at work for all people through research and prevention.

To receive NIOSH documents or information about occupational safety and health topics contact NIOSH at:

1-800-35-NIOSH (1-800-356-4674)

Fax: 1-513-533-8573

E-mail: pubstaft@cdc.gov
or visit the NIOSH web site at:
http://www.cdc.gov/niosh/hhe

SAFER • HEALTHIER • PEOPLE™